A Pocket Guide to Risk Assessment and Management in Mental Health

Risk assessment and risk management are top of every mental health organisation's agenda. This updated and expanded new edition provides an informative and practical guide to the process of undertaking a risk assessment, arriving at a risk formulation and developing a risk management plan.

Covering everything a practitioner may have to think about when undertaking risk assessments in an accessible, logical form, the second edition of *A Pocket Guide to Risk Assessment and Management in Mental Health* includes new and expanded content on: risk formulation; working in forensic settings; specific mental health disorders; models of suicide and self-harm; and triage. It features practice recommendations rooted in the latest theory and evidence base, clinical tip boxes, tables, diagrams and case examples, along with samples of authentic dialogue which demonstrate ways to formulate questions and think about complex problems with the person being assessed. A series of accompanying videos, professionally made and based on actual case studies, are available on a companion website, further illustrating key risk assessment and management skills.

This concise guidebook is designed for all mental health professionals, and professionals-in-training. It will also be a useful reference for all healthcare practitioners who regularly come into contact with people experiencing mental health problems.

Chris Hart is an independent nurse consultant, educator, facilitator and trainer, writer, film maker and academic. His specialist area of work now is risk assessment and risk management within the prison system, but he still works closely with mental health and non mental health NHS trusts and organisations to educate, train and develop staff in all aspects of risk assessment and management, as well as undertaking developmental work with senior nurses, clinicians and managers. He was previously a Senior Lecturer at Kingston University and St George's, University of London, UK and nurse consultant for South West London and St George's Mental Health NHS Trust.

A Pocket Guide to Risk Assessment and Management in Mental Health

Second Edition

Chris Hart

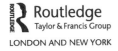

LONDON AND NEW YORK

Designed cover image: © Getty Images

Second edition published 2024
by Routledge
4 Park Square, Milton Park, Abingdon, Oxon, OX14 4RN

and by Routledge
605 Third Avenue, New York, NY 10158

Routledge is an imprint of the Taylor & Francis Group, an informa business

© 2024 Chris Hart

First edition published by Routledge 2014

British Library Cataloguing-in-Publication Data
A catalogue record for this book is available from the British Library

Library of Congress Cataloging-in-Publication Data
Names: Hart, Christopher, 1956- author.
Title: A pocket guide to risk assessment and management in mental health / Chris Hart.
Other titles: Pocket guide to risk assessment and management in mental health | Risk assessment and risk management
Description: Second edition. | Milton Park, Abingdon, Oxon ; New York, NY : Routledge, 2024. | Includes bibliographical references and index. |
Identifiers: LCCN 2023032552 | ISBN 9780367774813 (hardback) | ISBN 9780367774783 (paperback) | ISBN 9781003171614 (ebook)
Subjects: LCSH: Mental illness—Diagnosis—Handbooks, manuals, etc. | Mental illness—Treatment—Handbooks, manuals, etc. | Mental illness—Risk assessment—Handbooks, manuals, etc.
Classification: LCC RC454.4 .H368 2024 | DDC 616.89/075—dc23/eng/20230921
LC record available at https://lccn.loc.gov/2023032552

ISBN: 978-0-367-77481-3 (hbk)
ISBN: 978-0-367-77478-3 (pbk)
ISBN: 978-1-003-17161-4 (ebk)

DOI: 10.4324/9781003171614

Typeset in Sabon
by codeMantra

Access the Support Material: www.routledge.com/9780367774783

Contents

Figures

Tables

Boxes

Clinical examples

The accompanying films for the *Pocket Guide*

Several years ago the Head of Clinical Risk for the South West London and St George's Mental Health NHS Trust, Justin O'Brien, asked me to contribute to a unique project. It was to produce a series of films that would explore a range of risk assessment techniques in different scenarios, featuring interactions between mental health patients and clinicians.

The scripts were written by Justin and myself, sometimes with the help of colleagues working in the relevant clinical area. We then worked with professional actors provided by our great colleague, Cath Hamilton, a wonderful director in Andrew Calloway and their production crews to create films that could be used for education and training in this extremely complex area.

The films are all based on actual incidents or interactions with patients. Some include a part that demonstrates 'poor practice', often based on what had happened that had brought the incident to people's attention. Crucial to the making of the films was that they were credible and that the skills demonstrated in the 'good practice' section were achievable by the viewing audience.

The three films featured on the website to complement the text in the Pocket Guide came out of that work but are different in their subject matter. One focuses on the risk of suicide while the other explores a serious assault carried out on a clinician by a person who is psychotic. The first film has a section that shows poor practice, followed by a longer interview demonstrating how a relatively inexperienced nurse can carefully assess the person's risk in the context of his changed mental state. The second film explores danger to others, often thought to be 'unpredictable' by many clinicians working with people experiencing mental health problems. This film is staged very differently, showing a violent assault on a member of staff by a patient, then giving the viewer the opportunity to look for triggers and indications that it was likely to occur. The final part of the film features a lengthy interview with the patient, after the assault has occurred, during which his rationale for the assault emerges. The third film shows the complexities of working with a man, diagnosed with an emotionally unstable personality disorder, in a prison setting, but focuses on trying to understand how the impact of trauma affects a person and how to repond to that in a meangingful way.

Much of the material from Part 5 of the *Pocket Guide* links directly to the films. Although there is sample dialogue in the book, the films on the website demonstrate the techniques highlighted in the text in a wholly different way, with the viewer able to look for the non-verbal cues and the human dynamic between interviewer and interviewee. When Justin and I have used these films in teaching practice, course participants have always cited them as crucial learning. I hope that, in accessing them on the website and using the materials and exercises that go with them, you will find the films equally rewarding.

To access the Support Material please visit www.routledge.com/9780367774783.

Acknowledgements

The work in this book is completely influenced by the many gifted and learned clinicians I've worked with over the years. There are too many to mention, with a few notable exceptions. I would be negligent if I did not pay tribute to Justin O'Brien, a great friend, colleague and influence. Huge thanks also to Tony McGranaghan for his knowledge and experience, Vince Keaney, who originated all our work on risk assessment many years ago, and Ian Higgins, always a wise counsel and original thinker. I'm also grateful to have had the experience of working with a new generation of outstanding clinicians, teachers and collaborators in Jess Kelliher, Lily Harthill, Ritchie Veerapen, Rosemary Jambert-Gray, Laurie Dahl, Charlotte Clee and my old friend, Neil Lauchlan. I also want to thank Godfried Attafua, all my colleagues from Kingston University, the amazing nurses at the Orchid Mental Health Emergency Assessment Unit I worked with during the pandemic, Lewin Road's Assessment and Treatment Team, as well as the Liaison Psychiatry Team at St George's Hospital, especially the 'ever present' David Tracey. Many of their ideas and experiences are woven into the fabric of this book. Any mistakes are completely mine and for those I apologise in advance. This book is dedicated to the memory of my dear friend, colleague and 'brother', Harjinder Sehmi.

Introduction

About this guide

The principle aim of this *Pocket Guide* is to provide a brief, practical guide to the process of undertaking a risk assessment, arriving at a formulation and, from that, developing a risk management plan. There are those who suggest that it is impossible to predict risk behaviours, especially those involving violence, and that extreme events, such as homicide, can never be predicted. *The Pocket Guide*, however, works on the premise put forward by Maden (2007), that 'clinical risk assessment is consistently more accurate than chance', that while it may not be possible to predict someone will do a specific thing at a specific time, 'it is possible to make reasonable statements of probability and which factors will increase or decrease the risk of an event happening, the first step in managing that risk.

This book is designed to be used as an aide memoire and a prompt for clinicians in the workplace undertaking mental health risk assessments, including those working in non-mental health settings. However, it is also applicable as a foundation to risk assessment in specialist settings, such as forensic services and prisons. Although set out in clearly defined sections, it is important to remember that the practice of sitting down with someone and having this discussion will not necessarily reproduce the linear structure here. Indeed, one of the most important skills in undertaking risk assessments is the ability to 'go with' the person and their story, while retaining an internal structure that enables you to address all the pertinent issues and fully assess risk during the course of the interview.

This is not an academic text that will provide in depth information about suicide, self-harm or other risk behaviours – though there is an expanded discussion about the background to suicide and the section on dangerousness to others has been developed far more for this edition, along with a section dedicated to risk assessment in prison and forensic settings. This text is also not aimed at providing a theoretical discourse about risk assessment. Its practice recommendations are rooted in the latest theory and evidence base and there is also a reading list to provide additional information and more background theory. The main purpose of The *Pocket Guide* is to be used in clinical situations and be of practical help. In this context, the statistics and other information contained in Part 1 are not there to be viewed in isolation but integrated into the assessment process, helping you think about your patient in the wider context, applying known clinical risk indicators and statistical information to the individual whom you are assessing. For example, it is known that a man aged between 45 and 54, recently separated from his partner, unemployed and depressed is statistically at greater risk of experiencing suicidal ideas and acting upon them than a 25-year-old, newly-married man who is financially

DOI: 10.4324/9781003171614-1

stable with a successful career. This doesn't tell you that the 52-year-old man you are assessing will try and kill himself, but indicates there are specific risk factors to be taken into account which should inform your assessment.

While the *Pocket Guide* acknowledges the importance of other forms of risk, e.g. self neglect and vulnerability, it will focus mainly on risk to self, in the form of self-harm and suicide, and to others, in the form of violence and aggression. However, the principles can be applied to any area of risk assessment, e.g. falls in older people, vulnerable children etc.

It largely describes a collaborative process at all stages and stresses the need to look for the least restrictive options, yet also recognises that more restrictive and coercive approaches are sometimes necessary, particularly where concerns about safety are not shared between the assessor and person being assessed and the assessor's concerns to manage risk outweigh the requirements of a collaborative approach.

The *Pocket Guide* does not recommend or directly address the use of 'risk assessment tools', screening tools or other recognised tools for assessing such things as psychosis, depression and anxiety etc. There are several reasons for this: there will be guidance about how to use these with the tools themselves; different health organisations advocate the use of different tools and the tools themselves are, inevitably, of varying quality. Validated risk assessment or screening tools can be useful – and you may also use other assessment tools to assist in the risk assessment process – and their use is recommended where applicable. A significant advantage to using recognised and shared assessment tools, particularly those related to risk, is that they provide a common language, specific prompts, structure and force the clinician to ask questions, some of which might be quite difficult. However, a key factor in how they are used is that any tool is only as effective in assessing risk as the clinician using it and completing it should not distract from the overall process of assessment described here. Particularly, the person being interviewed should not feel they are being subjected to a 'tick box process'.

In the latter part of the book three particular case studies are used to illustrate different skills and particular areas of risk assessment (see boxes 1 and 2). The case studies cited here are based on actual people who were assessed and treated, but anonymised and adapted to maintain confidentiality. One focuses on a 35-year-old man who is experiencing suicidal thoughts in the community. Later, he is in discussion with a clinician after a suicide attempt, having ingested paracetamol tablets.[1] The second features a young man who is in hospital following a serious assault in the context of a psychotic disorder. The third focuses on a young woman who is hurting herself and experiencing suicidal ideas in the context of emotionally unstable personality disorder. In all these cases, the details of the individual's background rarely feature as prominent issues in the risk assessment itself as the conversation focuses on more immediate matters relating to the risks facing each person. However, it always provides a context for the current situation, particularly as it relates to trauma, and informs the clinician's responses.

You will note the reference to terms such as discussion and conversation in the above paragraph, while the overall task being described is that of a risk assessment. One of the skills the *Pocket Guide* will try and convey is the way in which an assessment can be conducted in a conversational way. While this may take slightly longer, it is likely to help the clinician develop a better relationship and elicit more information. Nonetheless, while there may be quite a distinct style, or 'voice', in the clinical examples within the *Pocket Guide* it is necessary to remember that every clinician needs to find their own voice and style rather than trying to remember a certain question or way of seeking information seen elsewhere.

The *Pocket Guide* is broken into five parts. Part 1 contains an overview of the risk assessment process and information related to risk assessment and risk management, including clinical risk indicators; Part 2 looks at different approaches to risk assessment and its general principles; Part 3 focuses on the process of, and skills needed for, undertaking a risk assessment; Part 4 concentrates on forensic risk assessment and management and Part 5 more generic risk management.

Finally, it is crucial to remind ourselves that, no matter how comprehensive and competent the assessment, risk can never be wholly eliminated. Rather, clinicians are engaged in risk minimisation in a dynamic process, with the level of engagement from the person involved in the assessment crucial to its outcome.

Box 1:   Case study – William

(*See clinical examples in Part 3, Undertaking a risk assessment*)

William is a 35-year-old man, recently separated from his partner, Kelly. This followed a difficult relationship in which he had become increasingly dependent on her, having been made redundant from his job in information technology. Since she left, he has struggled financially, with a recent cut in his benefits, and he is facing the prospect of losing his flat and having to move back to live with his mother.

His father died a year ago after a long illness. William found it difficult to come to terms with his loss. William's father, a quantity surveyor, was an important figure in his life, although their relationship wasn't particularly close, certainly not as warm as the relationship between William's brother and their father.

He has few friends and finds it hard to confide in others. He and his brother are close but William feels he always has to live up to his brother's achievements and never wants to appear 'weak' or unable to cope in his eyes. William has always experienced his mother as rather aloof and distant, though says they have a good relationship.

William has only taken cannabis on a few occasions, in his late teens. He has no history of alcohol abuse but, as he struggled to cope with mounting stress, began drinking more. When stressed, he says he cannot think clearly and feels the need to 'escape', finding both his feelings and the sense of 'crowded thoughts running in circles' too difficult to bear. He has stopped doing things like yoga, reading and going out, which he was doing until a few weeks before Kelly left.

Over the past five to six weeks he has had trouble getting off to sleep, He then wakes through the night. He feels tired in the morning and struggles to get out of bed. His appetite is diminished, he has trouble concentrating and is not enjoying things he used to. He can see no hope for the future and is convinced no one would miss him if he were no longer there. Unable to think clearly about things like paying his bills or looking after his flat, he can see no way out of his situation.

In the clinical examples, we meet William initially at home and then there are examples of discussion with him after he has been admitted to an acute psychiatric ward following an attempt to kill himself.

Box 2:   Case study – Oliver

(See clinical examples in Part 3, Undertaking a risk assessment)

Oliver is currently an inpatient on a forensic ward, having been transferred from a Psychiatric Intensive Care Unit. He was first admitted after assaulting a man in an apparently unprovoked attack in the street. Initially arrested by the police, he was thought to be psychotic and brought to hospital under Section 136 of the Mental Health Act. This was converted to a Section 3 after he was assessed. Now in his late thirties, he has a history of psychotic illness, with several lengthy admissions to hospital, always under the Mental Health Act. He was living in a hostel prior to this admission.

Oliver experienced his first psychotic episode three months after starting university. He had grown up in a small town in Scotland but moved to London with his mother after she left Oliver's father. He was six-years-old at the time. His father had been a successful commercial artist but suffered from a psychotic illness and was a heavy drinker, prone to violence when intoxicated. He died just before Oliver's 18th birthday. Oliver's mother had several partners after separating from her husband and Oliver claims one of them was violent and possibly sexually abusive. He now says that the same man has come to him in hospital and 'done things' though no one has visited.

Over the past five years, Oliver has become increasingly isolated. Once keen on cricket and football, he has lost interest in most things. He doesn't see his old friends and now rarely associates with anyone other than people he has met in hospital. He regularly smokes cannabis and skunk and has used a variety of other illicit drugs including cocaine, ecstasy and amphetamines. His illicit drug use is usually associated with a relapse in his mental state.

Oliver understands his experiences as being the result of him having special powers and being different to other people. However, he also feels vulnerable to what he terms 'being infected' by other people. His definition of this phenomena varies but he often describes it as people being able to put thoughts in his head, change the way he feels, both physically and emotionally, and control him in unpleasant ways. It has been observed that this phenomena usually seems to occur when he is feeling physically and psychologically aroused, anxious and/or angry. He will often ruminate on things that have been said and, when he is doing this, isolate himself and not communicate with others.

He has a history of violent assaults on other patients and members of staff while in hospital. This has always led to him being transferred to another ward but there has not been a detailed assessment to date about why he assaults others and there is not a clear risk formulation related to this.

Oliver has been described as experiencing paranoid delusions, auditory hallucinations, ideas of reference and thought insertion (see table 3.4). He currently presents as a risk to others on the ward, having made threats of physical violence to fellow patients and nurses, as well as punching and kicking another patient.

Cultural diversity

Risk assessment is never blind to issues of colour, race, ethnicity, gender or sexuality. While there may be specific risks more common to particular groups we have to consider the unique journey the individual patient has undertaken, to the point where they are sat in front of you, not just literally but through the course of their life.

NHS England's report 'The Five Year Forward View for Mental Health' comments that 'for many, especially Black, Asian, and minority ethnic people, their first experience of mental health care comes when they are detained under the Mental Health Act, often with police involvement, followed by a long stay in hospital' (Mental Health Taskforce, 2016, p. 3).

As clinicians, we should make a point of learning about the injustices and inequalities experienced by people from different racial and ethnic groups. People who define themselves as Black or Black British are:

- 50% more likely to be referred to mental health services by the police;
- 3–5 times more likely to be diagnosed with schizophrenia;
- four times more likely to be detained under the Mental Health Act than their White counterparts.

Of the 32 women detained under the Mental Health Act who died following restraint between 2012/13 and 2016/17, more than 20% were from the Black, Asian and Minority Ethnic (BAME) community (Hart, 2020).

As noted above, there can be an overlap between the criminal justice system and mental health services which might inadvertently impact upon people's attitudes to those working in the latter. The Lammy Review (2017), an independent review of the treatment of, and outcomes for BAME individuals in the Criminal Justice System conducted for the UK government, found Black people were:

- more than nine times as likely to be stopped and searched by police as White people;
- over three times as likely to be arrested as White people;
- more than five times as likely to have force used against them by police as White people.

A quarter of the prison population comes from BAME backgrounds, despite representing just 14% of the population. In young offenders institutions, this increases to 50%.

Such experiences sit in the consciousness of communities, as do everyday discriminations and slights, whether conscious or unconscious, that the person may have experienced within the healthcare system. There is also research that suggests Black adults' experience of discrimination may be a more serious predictor of suicide risk than depression and non-discriminatory risk factors (Ducharme and Ross, 2022).

There is nothing the clinician can do to fix this in one session, particularly if it is intense and focuses on serious issues about the person's safety. However, sensitivity to the person's experiences and perceptions are essential and an integral part of their treatment.

It isn't possible to detail all the variations in cultural diversity that could impact on a risk assessment. These have to be an essential part of your assessment. If you are assessing someone about whose culture you have little understanding, it is important to endeavour to find out any information that will help you arrive at a clear formulation and to make clear, safe clinical decisions. Equally, if language is a barrier, you should seek the assistance of a professional interpreter (it is inadvisable to use a carer/friend or to find someone 'who speaks the language' to undertake such a complex task unless conducting an emergency assessment with no opportunity to arrange the assistance of an interpreter).

Gender and sexuality

Again, it isn't possible to explore in detail the variety of gender issues relevant to the risk assessment process within the space of the *Pocket Guide*, nor those related to sexual orientation. It's important, always, to remember that people from the LGTBQ+ community are at greater risk of self-harm and suicide than the general population. In Part 1 there are detailed statistics that delineate risks for different groups and there will be occasional references to specific risk factors, e.g. sexual abuse and its relationship to self-harm, transgender and self-harm. Most sections of the *Pocket Guide* will help you think about accessing specific risks and exploring different risk indicators through the assessment process with a view to making that assessment completely relevant to the individual, regardless of gender or sexual orientation. Part of this is checking out how the person wants to be addressed while also thinking about your gender as the person assessing the patient. Are they comfortable with you? Are there reasons they might find it challenging to talk to you about their sexuality, gender or issues of abuse? Is it possible to have someone the person will be more comfortable with conduct the assessment? This obviously isn't always possible, but asking these questions and being sensitive to the issues may help the person feel more comfortable.

Models of care

Many mental health teams now have strict criteria for patients for whom they will provide a service. This also means having exclusion criteria. Patients can be assessed and declined a service from a particular team even though that might increase the risk. The team may decline to see the person without any assessment. It's therefore important to think about how that is routinely managed, including any process for referring the person on. What do you tell the patient? How is it communicated? Has any of this changed the risk?

If it is your team receiving the referral and commencing work with the person, remember that a new assessment of risk is always required.

A note about terminology

Different terms are used in any number of different settings and texts for and about the people who use or come into contact with mental health services. The most important – and simple – element to communicate about the assessment process is that it is an exchange between people. It will always be easier if the clinician remembers that.

While there are different rationales for preferring each term, I shall talk about people, the person and individual in most cases but use the term patient when necessary as there is evidence that people using mental health services prefer to be described as patients rather than clients, service users or customers (Barker, 2003; Simmons et al., 2010; McGuire-Sneickus et al., 2003).

Note

1 In each clinical example, reference is made only to a 'clinician'. This is because the skills and risk assessments illustrated here could be conducted by any variety of mental health and non-mental health clinicians, rather than just psychiatrists or mental health nurses.

References

Barker, P. (2003) *Assessment in Practice*. In Barker, P. (ed.) *Psychiatric and Mental Health Nursing: The craft of caring*. London: Hodder Arnold.

Ducharme, J. and Ross, J. (2022) What We Misunderstand About Suicide Among Black Americans. *Time*, February 4.

Hart, C. (2020) We Can Talk About How Things Can Be Different. *Nursing Times Opinion*, August 13. www.nursingtimes.net.

McGuire-Sneickus, R., McCabe, R. and Preibe, S. (2003) Patient, Client or Service User? A survey of patient preferences in dress and address of six mental health professions. *Psychiatric Bulletin*, 27, 305–308.

Simmons P., Hawley C.J., Gale, T.M. and Sivakumaram, T. (2010) Service user, patient, client, user or survivor: describing recipients of mental health services. *The Psychiatrist*, 34, 20–23.

The Lammy Review (2017) https://www.gov.uk/government/publications/lammy-review-final-report.

Part 1
Risk assessment; an overview

Introduction

Assessment, in the context of mental health, refers to the process of gathering and analysing information from multiple and diverse sources, including a semi-structured interview with the person concerned, in order to develop an understanding, and evaluation, of a possible mental health problem (see Box 3 below).

It is the fundamental starting point for any process of care. Assessment determines the clinician's understanding of the issues the patient wishes to address, as well as the clinician's concerns about the person, which that person may not share. Moreover, it presents an opportunity to listen to the person's story. This, with the exploration of strengths, coping strategies, problems and/or needs is a key part of establishing a rapport with the person, which is essential when risk needs to be assessed. Considering all elements of risk is a core part of the overall assessment process.

Risk is a *neutral* occurrence but with an implied possibility of loss or hazard. In the context of mental health, risk has been described as:

> The likelihood of behaviour (or situations) that may be harmful or beneficial to oneself or to others. Risk assessment involves analysing potential outcomes of this behaviour (or situation); and risk management involves devising a care plan to minimise harmful behaviour and maximise beneficial behaviour.
>
> (Callaghan and Waldcock, 2006)

Appleby et al. (2018) defined it as:

> Risk assessment combines consideration of psychological and social factors as part of a comprehensive review to capture patient care needs, and to assess their risk of harm to themselves or others.

The *Pocket Guide* works on the basis that it is far more effective to use discussion in the form of a semi-structured interview as the basis for the clinician's approach rather than a 'checklist approach' (Alderdice et al., 2010). It also recognises that some people who either go on to harm themselves or others or are experiencing ideas about risk behaviours, e.g. attempting suicide, will verbally deny them, thus necessitating the very rigorous,

DOI: 10.4324/9781003171614-2

inquisitive and holistic methodology detailed here. Above all, it should be remembered that risk is:

- a dynamic process – different elements can change, altering the risks and their impact on the patient. Indeed, as soon as a clinician intervenes through the process of an assessment, risk is affected. We would hope it begins to minimise it but there is the possibility that, in addressing one risk, another arises (see below);
- context dependent – what is 'risky' in one context may not be in another.

Most importantly, as has already been emphasised, we must remember that no matter how good the risk assessment, risk cannot be eliminated, only minimised. Risk behaviours are influenced by:

- the situation the person finds themselves in;
- their personal background;
- their own psychopathology;
- a range of clinical risk factors (see 'Organisational issues and risk assessment and risk management' and 'Risk of suicide and self-harm', pages 13 and 16);
- the context in which the person is acting.

Box 3:   The principles of risk assessment

- Gathering and analysing information;
- taking a rigorous approach – involving the multi-disciplinary team wherever possible;
- matching the time to the potential seriousness of the situation or using the available time to gather the essential information;
- adopting as collaborative an approach as possible;
- communicating the risk effectively and clearly;
- using a shared model understood by all members of the clinical team and communicated to potential referrers.

Key issues to determine from a risk assessment

Interviewing the patient and significant others offers the opportunity to gather key information. Past risk behaviours and risk history are good indicators of current risk. When looking at past incidents, consider the nature of the incident specifically and accurately. For example, what harm was caused? What were the background circumstances of the incident? Who suffered harm? What risk factors were present at the time? It is also important to explore what was going on in the patient's life at the time.

As well as identifying all possible risks, i.e. to the person themselves and/or others, it is essential to have determined the following at the conclusion of even a brief risk assessment (see also Table 1.1).

Recentness

How recent was the risk event? Where multiple incidents have occurred the current risk must be seen as greater than if it were isolated. However, it is vital to review the current situation in the context of the entire risk history for the person you're with, even if the last incident was a considerable time ago or the circumstances initially appear to be different.

Immediacy

Try to establish how immediate the risk is. If there doesn't appear to be any current risk, what would change to make *potential* risks *actual* risks or, if recent risks are no longer current, what has changed to bring this about?

Severity

The more serious the potential consequences of an incident, the more robust you will need to be in addressing it, even if the person is reluctant to engage, tries to assure you there is no longer any risk or other clinicians have not appeared concerned.

Patterns

When undertaking the assessment you should be looking for common patterns that lead to an incident occurring, including anything in the person's relapse profile or risk history.

Background

Was there trauma experienced by the person as a child? This may have impacted on their resilience as an adult. Previous exposure to others' suicide – not just in their family – makes it more likely the person will be vulnerable to suicide themselves. Impulsivity, interpersonal stressors and physical illness and/or chronic pain can all increase the risk of suicide.

Thinking

Questions can be framed to explore the way in which the person thinks, looking for things like:

- cognitive rigidity;
- difficulty solving problems;
- seeking perfection but experiencing a sense of failure when it can't be achieved;
- attentional bias – seeing only the negative and unable to remember successes;
- reasons for living;
- ruminations, and their content.

Emotions

Assessing the overall level of *distress* is important in thinking about how much control the person is able to exercise in keeping themselves safe. This is not necessarily going to be visible or obvious but is about how the person feels. Other issues to consider are whether or not the person feels:

* a burden on others;
* defeated and/or trapped;
* alone or alienated;
* no longer afraid of hurting themselves or even death;
* most important, hopeless.

Intent

Rather than accepting the actual consequences of the person's actions, which may not have been particularly harmful, it is essential to explore their intent.

For example:

* Although an overdose of the actual medication taken could not have been lethal, the person may not have known this and still intended to end their life by taking it.
* Equally, a potentially lethal action may have been undertaken without the person realising how dangerous it actually was or any intention to end their life, e.g. someone taking 20 paracetamol tablets thinking it will put them to sleep for a while and not understanding this could kill them.
* An individual may have been prevented from harming someone else, or not inflicted significant harm in an assault. However, this cannot be presumed to reveal the person's actual intent. Explore thoroughly what they would have done had the opportunity been there to complete the assault uninterrupted, or, now they have been thwarted, what they would do if they got another opportunity. Moreover, if there is any intention to harm a specific individual, that person should be informed at the earliest opportunity and, if appropriate, the police should also be informed.
* Therefore, explore:
  * What did the person want to achieve with their actions?
  * What did they expect to happen?
  * If it was an attempt to end their life, was that their intention or did they act with the intention of escaping their situation and ending their life seemed the only way to achieve that?
* Having survived, how do they feel now?
* Would they want to try again – remembering that the person who has attempted suicide and regrets surviving is very likely to make a further attempt.
* If they wanted to die and now say they don't, what has changed?

Current intent is one of the strongest indicators of future behaviour.

Frequency

The more frequent the incidents, the greater the risk and the more robust the assessor needs to be in addressing them. Is the intensity and dangerousness of the behaviours escalating? Are the gaps between incidents narrowing? If so, how has the risk management plan been adapted to this?

Warning signs

How would anyone know things were getting worse? What would the person be saying and/or doing? What would others see? Crucially, would the person let people know if things were deteriorating?

Planning

The level of planning by the patient prior to carrying out a behaviour is an indicator of both the intent and the broader elements of risk to be managed and should be explored thoroughly, including:

- When did the person first start thinking about doing something harmful to themselves or others?
- What options did they consider for doing this?
- How did they rule things out and come to their final choice of means of acting?
- When did this become a 'plan' that they knew they would act on?
- How many things had to be done to put the plan into action, for example, looking on internet sites for information about potential lethality, buying tablets or obtaining a specific weapon, waiting for the opportunity to be alone, luring a victim to a specific place?
- Had other things been done, e.g. the person putting their affairs in order, getting pets looked after, writing letters for loved ones?
- Had the person had to actively deceive others to carry out the plan, e.g. concealing things, telling them they were going to be doing something else, going somewhere else that would have appeared to be safe?
- How long was the plan in place before acted upon?
- Was there anything specific that led the person to initiate the plan at the time they did?

Level of collaboration

How likely is the person to work with any risk management plan? How is the individual's willingness to collaborate influenced by issues such as capacity, insight/awareness and attitude to treatment?

How robustly have you been able to test out the person's willingness to collaborate, e.g. by a mental capacity assessment, whether or not the person will attend appointments or give you access to their premises, whether they are keeping to agreed care plans, offering information, allowing you opportunities to talk to family and/or carers?

Table 1.1 Key issues to identify during a risk assessment

Who	is the person(s) at risk?
What	are the specific risk(s)? Name each risk identified.
When	is the person at risk, e.g. now? In the future – what would change to increase or minimise the risk? If the person was assessed as previously being at risk but is not now – *what has changed?* Are there changes to the risk during the course of the day, e.g. is the person more at risk at night, if they can't sleep, or if left alone during the day?
Where	is the risk behaviour most likely to be enacted? Is the person safe in their current environment? Do they need to be in a more restrictive environment or seen more frequently?
Why	is the person currently vulnerable to these risks?
How	would the person harm themselves or others? Do they have a specific plan or might they act opportunistically? Are they impulsive or methodical?

WHAT IS THE PLAN TO ADDRESS EACH CURRENT AND POTENTIAL RISK?
Has it been documented? Has it been communicated?

Key clinical tip – the *What if?* question

A comprehensive risk assessment carefully considers the "What if?" questions, e.g. what if something happens that might affect the risk, what would the person do in certain situations? If this highlights potential, as opposed to actual, risk it should lead to **contingency planning** to address those potential situations.

Organisational issues and risk assessment and risk management

The *Pocket Guide* cannot address team functioning and organisation in depth but it is worth considering some key organisational, team and individual issues that increase the effectiveness of risk assessment and management – and, conversely, can cause serious problems if ignored.

Organisational factors that can undermine effective risk assessment and risk management

A crucial starting point for any healthcare organisation is to have coherent and robust policies both for risk assessment and risk management that reflect the real, lived experience of staff engaged in work where they will be undertaking these tasks, e.g. lone working, home visits. These should be easily accessible and user friendly, i.e. readable, not full of jargon and as brief as possible.

Organisations should, however, not make the mistake of thinking that having a good policy in place means it has fulfilled its responsibilities and all will be well. There should be a confidence borne out of experience that the policies are effective in influencing practice and are helpful to staff in their clinical practice.

This should be supported by clinical governance structures that effectively address issues of risk and disseminate learning, not just from serious incidents and near misses but also good practice, with reflective practice and clinical supervision available to all staff.

Other issues include:

- resolving conflicting service demands e.g. waiting times for admissions/bed pressures;
- addressing staffing shortages or lack of resources, even if this means service or team re-organisation;
- caseloads have to be set at a level that allows sufficient time for good practice. If this is not the case, managers need to think about what they will do to mitigate the clinical risk;
- models of care and thinking *must* accommodate the patient's needs and not exclude patients/moving people from one service or team to another for organisational rather than clinical reasons.

Perhaps most importantly, clinicians cannot let any lack of resource influence the assessment process or dictate a risk management plan. Always, the optimal risk management plan must be identified and recorded, even if that then has to be adapted to accommodate the realities of the team's available resource.

Team factors that can undermine effective risk assessment and risk management

- Systematic risk assessment not undertaken;
- care plans either not being used or not used consistently;
- risk indicators denied or minimised by the group;
- clinical responsibility not clearly defined or transferred appropriately;
- poor communication internally and with other agencies;
- poor liaison with other agencies;
- inadequate support to clinicians managing patients with immediate risk.

Individual factors that can undermine effective risk assessment and risk management

- The knowledge, experience, capability and attitudes of the clinician;
- workload, time and difficulty responding to pressures from colleagues and/or referrers;
- the emotional and psychological capacity to manage difficult work at any one time.

It is important to recognise that all of these factors will vary over time and be affected by a variety of internal and external influences (Hart, 2006).

Addressing individual and structural deficits

Key principles

1. Building productive, well managed and well led teams that work together is crucial.
2. Those with the responsibility to manage risk must also have the authority to make decisions.
3. Senior clinicians and managers need to understand the experience of frontline staff on inpatient units and respond to it, e.g. listening to dynamic risk changes, views on prescribing, levels of observation etc.

Other factors

1. Provide skill-based training and education programmes that integrate theory with the realities of practice.
2. Provide individual and team clinical supervision that addresses caseloads/patient allocation at least monthly, giving staff safe forums for thinking and talking about patients.
3. Develop work practices that increase emotional intelligence.
4. Resources have to be made available to manage risk – there is a huge disincentive on clinicians to 'reveal' risk if they are expected to manage it without the necessary support and resource.
5. Barriers to rapid assessment have to be removed.
6. Accessible and responsive services have to be more than an aspiration or slogan.
7. Services should be designed with cohesive risk management as a core principle and foundation of the service.
8. The culture of unnecessarily saying 'No' to referrers has to be eradicated.
9. Develop organisational models that support risk assessment.
10. Have defined clinical models of care for inpatient units.
11. Develop strong relational management – improve staff-management relations and staff input into decision making.
12. Bridge the gap between the managerial/business ideology and clinical culture (Harrison and Hart, 2006).
13. Individual clinicians have a responsibility to:

   - seek help and/or advice when they need it;
   - make sure they have the knowledge and skills required for the work they are asked to do and highlight their training needs if necessary;
   - not let themselves be pressured into undertaking a risk assessment if they are aware they are unable to complete it adequately.

Common findings from inquiries

If any of the factors listed in Box 4 are present in a case with which you are working, they should alert you to potentially serious problems, a conversation in the team and a plan drawn up to address them.

Box 4:   Frequent findings from inquiries into suicide and homicide

- Confusion over diagnosis.
- Risk incidents being viewed in isolation.
- Delays or inappropriate responses.
- Poor record keeping.
- Poor inter-agency co-ordination.
- Poor communication between agencies.
- Not acknowledging family/carer concerns.
- Lack of clarity about confidentiality.

- Training specific to risk is lacking.
- Non-compliance with treatment plans not being addressed when this is known to be a risk factor.
- Lack of face to face contact with the patient (Appleby et al., 2006).

Risk of suicide and self-harm

Key definitions

There are no universally agreed definitions for suicide and what is sometimes termed parasuicide. The fifth edition of the *Diagnostic and Statistical Manual of Mental Disorders* (2013) describes two types of self-harming behaviour in non-suicidal self injury and suicidal behaviour disorder. The reality of understanding the acts described below is that they are often far more complex than these definitions allow. However, in order to develop a broad understanding, unambiguous and widely understood terms are useful.

Self-harm

This has been described as a non-fatal act, carried out intentionally to inflict harm, in the form of an acute episode of behaviour by an individual with variable motivation (Gelder et al., Hawton et al. (2013) described it as intentional acts of self poisoning or self injury irrespective of the type of motivation or degree of suicidal intent.

Attempted suicide

This involves self injurious behaviour with varying degrees of suicidal intent with a non-fatal outcome.

Parasuicide

Although commonly used, this is a term that often confuses attempted suicide, self-harm and 'a cry for help'. Hawton (2005), an internationally recognised expert on the subject, describes it as 'non fatal deliberate self-harm', though most contemporary writers would not now include the term 'deliberate'.

Suicide

This is a self inflicted act, causing one's own death. Suicide may be direct or indirect. There will be varying degrees of suicidal intent.

Suicide is a *direct act* when an individual takes an action that leads to the loss of their own life, e.g. by self poisoning or hanging, either as an end to be attained, i.e. to be dead, or as a means to another end, such as when a person ends their life to escape unbearable feelings or a particular situation, or can see no other solution to a set of problems.

Suicide has been described as an *indirect act* when one does not do what is necessary to escape death, such as leaving a burning building, but this would not meet a legal definition.

Self-harm

The phrase 'self-harm' is used to describe a range of things that people do to themselves in an intentional and often hidden way. The act can be planned or impulsive. It can involve:

- cutting;
- burning;
- scalding;
- banging or scratching one's own body;
- breaking bones;
- hair pulling;
- swallowing poisonous substances or objects, including prescribed medication and illicit drugs;
- hanging;
- strangulation;
- food refusal (although there are complex factors influencing this);
- mutilation of parts of the body, including inserting objects;
- interfering with wound healing;
- some forms of self neglect.

It's possible to add in things like misuse of alcohol and drugs (in some cases these are consciously used as a form of self-harm) and, of course, there are lots of lifestyle choices that are harmful. However, the key thing to consider is whether or not the overriding intention of the act is for the person to harm themselves.

Motives for self-harm

These will be highly personal or individual and do not necessarily sit within medicalised or biological models (see Table 1.2). Motives can include:

- A release of tension, frustration or distress;
- to feel and/or regain control;
- releasing 'bad' feelings;
- self punishment;
- to assuage feelings of guilt;
- an incapacity to understand and manage painful feelings;
- as a means of expressing emotional pain;
- to influence others (sometimes referred to as 'instrumental' self-harm);
- providing a feeling of 'wellness', linked to the possible release of endorphins and utilisation of the neurotransmitter, serotonin.

The person who is highly aroused may describe themselves as feeling:

- stressed;
- overwhelmed;
- unable to cope;
- hypersensitive.

Conversely, and less common, those in a dissociated state may describe themselves as feeling:

- numb;
- empty;
- 'lost';
- disconnected;
- unreal (see Figure 1.1).

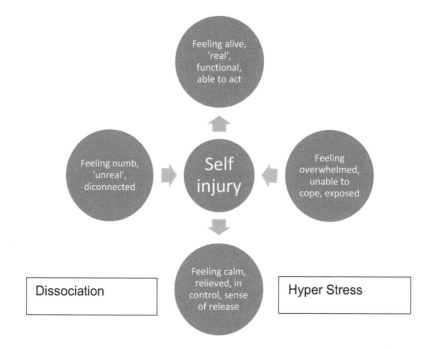

Figure 1.1 Psychological states and potential self harm

Source: APMS 2016, NHS Digital. Copyright 2016, Health and Social Care Information Centre

Repeated self-harm is often associated with the desire to manage unbearable psychic pain and/or unbearable situations and can include the wish to die (Hjelmeland et al., 2002; O'Connor et al., 2009). The physical pain or discomfort that stems from the act can provide distraction and/or a sense of relief. People self-harming may be confused about their motives or those motives not really known to them, while the motives for self-harm can change over time and even become habitual (Horne and Csipke, 2009).

Table 1.2 Methods and reasons for self-harming, by sex

Adults who reported in self-completion having ever self-harmed			*2014*
		Sex	
Self-reported method and reason for self-harming	Male	Female	Total
	per cent	per cent	per cent
Method of self-harming			
Cut self	66.2	77.0	73.1
Burned self	16.8	6.5	10.2
Swallowed something	17.1	11.9	13.8
Harmed self in other way	32.2	27.4	29.1
Reasons harmed self			
To draw attention	23.8	35.0	31.0
To relieve unpleasant feelings	66.8	82.1	76.7

Source: APMS 2016, NHS Digital. Copyright 2016, Health and Social Care Information Centre

Ruminations, distress and self-harm – the Emotional Cascade model

We often look at a complex array of external triggers, e.g. the loss of a relationship, financial hardship, bullying etc. However, these external events need an internal layer to provoke self-harm. This seems to come in the form of rumination, a process of reflection and brooding which focuses on negative feelings or emotions and leads to a strong negative emotional state. Negative emotional stimuli can attract the already distressed person's attention and increase their rumination.

This then progressively exacerbates the negative emotional state, weakening the person's ability to turn their attention away from it, creating an emotional cascade that becomes unbearable. Difficult to interrupt by functional or harmless means, this cycle often prompts intense behaviours to regulate their emotions and distract themselves from their rumination, including self-harm but also aggression and/or violence, substance misuse and even suicide (Selby and Joiner, 2009; Gardner et al., 2014).

Self-harm and the Cry of Pain model

More often identified as a means of understanding suicidal behaviour, the Cry of Pain Model asserts that self-harming behaviours are a result of feeling trapped in a stressful situation from which there is a perception of no escape or rescue (Williams and Pollock, 2001). Four key predictors will be present for self-harm:

1. stress;
2. the perception of defeat;
3. the perception of entrapment, fuelled by a perception of events and feelings being outside the person's control;
4. the perception that there is no possibility of 'escaping' the situation, or being 'rescued', often fuelled by poorer social support.

Lower levels of depression, a sense of entrapment and deficits in coping strategies are more predictive of self-harm. When these are higher, suicidal behaviour is more likely.

Self-harm statistics

It is important to note that, as with clinical risk indicators (see the 'Clinical Risk Indicators' section, page 39), the statistics in this section cannot be seen as reliable predictors of individual behaviour. However, they are included here for two reasons.

Firstly, they serve as a reminder of the vulnerability of particular client groups with whom we often feel so familiar that it is easy to underestimate or overlook the risk levels. Secondly, it is important to recognise that risk factors vary across age, gender and for different groups in society.

For example, self-harm among older people has a distinct and different profile, with suicidal intent often far more prominent (Dennis et al., 2007). One piece of research into young people and self-harm found different forms of self-harm may indicate different intent. Only 40 per cent of those who had cut themselves had wanted to die, while 66 per cent who self poisoned had sought death (Alderdice, 2010). Reasons for self-harm among South Asian women will often be very different from White European women (Bhugra and Desai, 2002).

Estimates of the numbers of people who self-harm in the UK vary. It is recognised that people who self-harm may not seek medical treatment for their injury or after self poisoning. Though some will tell a medical or mental health clinician, that may not be collated into any form of nationally recognised statistical base. However, Horrocks and House (2002) have estimated there are 400,000 episodes per year and people with mental health problems are 20 times more likely to self-harm than the general population.

NHS Digital (2019) cite self-harm as the cause for at least 114,000 general hospital presentations in 2018–2019, with over 20,000 of those being people aged 15–19. However, Clements et al. (2016) noted 'there was a consistent under estimation of presentations for self-harm by Hospital Episode Statistics emergency department data', and the figure was more likely to be 200,000 plus presentations for self-harm to emergency departments each year, with 20 per cent of those people re-presenting to the department within a year. House and Owens (2020) suggest it is reasonable to estimate that as many as 4 million people attended UK hospitals between 1994 and 2019 following an episode of self-harm, 'with 30,000 of those attendances being followed by suicide within 12 months'.

Repetition of self-harm increases the risk of suicide and at least 15–25 per cent repeat an act of self-harm within a year of their previous incident. Risk of repetition is greatest within the first few weeks of the earlier act and repetition increases the risk of eventual suicide (Hawton, 2005; Zahl and Hawton, 2004).

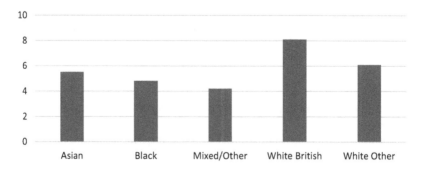

Figure 1.2 Percentage of people aged 16 years and over who had self harmed, by ethnicity

Source: APMS 2016, NHS Digital. Copyright 2016, Health and Social Care Information Centre

Adults aged 16 and over and self-harm

As seen in Table 1.3, *The Adult Psychiatric Morbidity Survey*[i] (2016) found 'the overall rate of self-harm in the adult population (7.3 per cent) was comparable to that for suicide attempt (6.7 per cent)'. Rates among women were higher at 8.9 per cent, with men at 5.7 per cent but the age gradient was far more dramatic.

Table 1.3 Prevalence of self-harm by age and sex

Age	16–24	25–34	35–44	45–54	55–64	65–74	75 +	All
	per cent	per cent	per cent	per cent	per cent	per cent	per cent	per cent
Men	9.7	10.9	6.6	3.3	3.3	2.0	-	5.7
Women	25.7	13.2	9.2	5.0	5.0	1.8	0.6	8.9
All adults	17.5	12.1	7.9	4.1	4.1	1.9	0.3	7.3

Source: APMS 2016, NHS Digital. Copyright 2016, Health and Social Care Information Centre

Groups experiencing a greater risk of self-harm include:

- people who have experienced physical, emotional or sexual abuse during childhood;
- people who have experienced serious psychological and/or physical trauma – trauma being defined as 'a disordered psychic or behavioural state resulting from severe mental or emotional stress or physical injury';
- LGBTQ+ people, who seem to be more likely to self-harm, as well as other minority groups discriminated against by society (RCP, 2006);
- people with pervasive developmental disabilities such as autism will often self-harm;
- people who are depressed or have other significant mental health problems – those with mental health problems are 20 times more likely to self-harm than people in the general population;
- people dependent on drugs or alcohol;
- those facing major life problems or living in very stressful circumstances at times they feel particularly vulnerable;
- veterans;
- asylum seekers.

Young people and self-harm

Young women are most likely to self-harm, though the number of young men who self-harm is increasing. There was a tripling in poisonings of paracetamol and antidepressants among 10–24 year-olds between 1998 and 2014 and it has been estimated that 7–14 per cent of adolescents will self-harm at some time in their life, with a common factor being feelings of helplessness or powerlessness.

A YouGov poll from 2018 found 36 per cent of 16–25 year-olds in Britain had self-harmed at some point in their lives. The Children's Society (2018) analysed a survey of 11,000 14-year-olds and found that:

- as many as 1 in 10 people may self-harm at some time in their life;
- nearly 25 per cent of girls and nearly 10 per cent of boys had self-harmed in a year;
- as many as 76,000 girls and 33,000 boys aged 14 may be self-harming.

Sexual abuse and self-harm

- The impact of the experience of childhood abuse on adult self-harm is now well established, as is its link with suicidal behaviour, particularly among women (Bebbington et al., 2009).
- Where abuse is repeated and sexual abuse was by a member of the immediate family, there is a stronger association with suicide attempts (Brezo et al., 2008).
- There is a likelihood of increased risk of self-harm in people with a history of childhood sexual abuse, particularly if the abuse is perpetrated over a long period, the victim knows the perpetrator and forced penetration was used (Cutliffe, 2005).

The issue of sexual abuse is important, as can be seen, and could potentially be spoken about by someone during a risk assessment, particularly if the presenting problem is one of self-harm or suicide. Whether or not it is best to explore this in a risk assessment needs careful consideration (see clinical example 10, page 126).

Prognosis

All these statistics should alert clinicians to the huge risks associated with people who present and re-present with self-harm about whom it is often felt there is no serious suicide risk, that the person 'isn't serious' or that every presentation is the same and therefore doesn't merit a proper assessment.

Every time someone presents with self-harm the situation may have changed and there may be a significant risk of them going on to attempt suicide or, indeed, this may have been an occasion when the act was one of suicidal intent rather than self-harm.

The commonly expressed view that people who self-harm are either 'not serious' or will not go on to kill themselves is *not* borne out by the evidence. The prognosis following an episode of self-harm is poor:

- the rate of completed suicide in people who have self-harmed in the previous year is 100 times that of the general population;
- suicide rates are highest within the first six months after the index self-harm incident;
- 1 in 50 patients who attend hospital after self-harm will die by suicide within one year and one in 15 within nine years (Owens, Horrocks and House, 2002);
- more than 50 per cent of people who die by suicide have self-harmed, 15 per cent within the previous year (Gairin, House and Owens, 2003).

However, the risk of self-harm escalating, either to further self-harm attempts or suicide attempts, can be offset by offering a psychosocial assessment, as recommended in the NICE Guidelines (2004). A study of people presenting with self-harm to Emergency Departments found that a psychosocial assessment reduced the risk of a single repeat episode by 51 per cent in individuals without a history of psychiatric treatment and by 26 per cent in individuals with a history of psychiatric treatment. For those people with a repetition of up to five episodes, a psychosocial assessment decreased the risk of a further episode by 13 per cent (Bergen et al., 2010).

Suicide

The myths

- "If someone is really serious, they'd go away and do it."
- "People who tell you they're going to kill themselves are never going to do it."
- "If someone is determined to kill themselves, there's nothing you can do to stop them."
- "The people who really want to die are never going to tell anyone."

These kinds of statements are, unfortunately, not uncommon among healthcare professionals and inaccurate and dangerous if they influence clinicians' behaviour towards people at risk. They often reflect negative attitudes towards people presenting with self-harm and suicide as described at least as far back as the seminal article, 'Normal Rubbish: deviant patients in casualty' (1979), in which one doctor was quoted as saying, "I think it's all so unnecessary, you know, if you are going to do the job (end your life), do it properly, don't bother us!"

In fact, most people who complete the act of suicide will have sought help, told someone they were thinking about it or at least dropped hints. Pearson et al. (2009) found that 91 per cent of individuals had seen their GP at least once in the year before death, with an average of seven consultations, almost double the general population rate.

A systematic review of the literature on contact with primary care and mental health services prior to suicide found:

> Contact with primary health care was highest in the year prior to suicide with an average contact rate of 80 per cent. At one month [prior to death], the average rate was 44 per cent. The lifetime contact rate for mental health care was 57 per cent, and 31 per cent in the final 12 months.
>
> (Stene-Larsen and Reneflot, 2017)

There is also evidence people who are serious about suicide but prevented from acting upon their plans rarely go on to end their life. In August 1937, less than two months after it opened, World War One veteran Harold Wobber stepped onto San Francisco's Golden Gate Bridge and history. Wobber turned to a stranger on the walkway and said, "This is as far as I go, " then jumped to his death. He was the first of over 1,500 people to end their life on the bridge – along with hundreds more who died unseen or unreported (Guthmann, 2005). Yet a study by suicidologist Richard Seiden (1978) discovered only six percent of 515 people prevented from jumping off the bridge between 1937 and 1971 went on to kill themselves.

Moreover, it is impossible to quantify how many lives have been saved without the person who made the vital difference knowing the impact they've had.

There are obvious examples: the prison officer who cuts a prisoner's ligature and stops him hanging himself, the paramedic or police officer who talks someone down from jumping off a bridge, the nurse who finds someone cutting themselves and intervenes. Yet every clinician reading this may well have done or said *something* that made a difference to someone preparing or seriously thinking of ending their life. It might have been giving that person an extra few minutes, which allowed them to challenge their own thoughts, asking the questions that enable them to tell you how they are really feeling and what they're contemplating, a small act of kindness that distracts them from their rumination.

One example is that of Jonny Benjamin. He has described how, soon after being diagnosed with schizoaffective disorder, feeling hopeless and suicidal and recently discharged from a psychiatric hospital, he was "in [his] own world standing at the edge of [Waterloo] bridge, trying to find the right point to jump". Neil Laybourn, a complete stranger, noticed him and started talking to him. "When he came along it burst the bubble of that world I was in. I felt like I could talk to him." Benjamin said it was Laybourn's compassion and simple words that affected him. Laybourn asked Benjamin to step back and go for a coffee and a chat with him. Benjamin eventually climbed down (Siddique, 2014).[ii]

Equally, strategic interventions, such as introducing compassionate, supportive and high quality psychosocial interventions for people presenting to Emergency Departments following an episode of self-harm or a suicide attempt, reduce the numbers going on to self-harm and complete suicide (Guthrie et al., 2001; Carter et al., 2016; Quinliven et al., 2021), and even reducing the number of paracetamol tablets that can be purchased from one shop reduced the number of people dying by paracetamol overdose.

The simple lesson of all these things is that the more knowledgeable and skilled the clinician, the more able they are to act with compassion and exercise the emotional labour to support their knowledge and skills, the more likely they are to be successful in helping the person remain safe and alive.

Socio-economic reasons for suicide: what is known

The relationship between self-harm and suicide is complex. Although acts of self-harm and apparent suicide attempts do not necessarily involve an intention to die, there is a strong association between self-harm, attempted suicide and subsequent death by suicide.

Equally, the reasons why people end their life, and when and how they make the decision to do so are extremely complex. While this is a guide to the practical assessment and management of clinical risk, a brief pause to consider some of the underlying factors might help us develop a greater understanding of the complexities of this process and what we're looking for in assessments. It becomes immediately apparent that while mental disorders are the most significant factor in suicide there are others, often affecting huge groups of people at the same time, that have to be considered.

In the 22 years following the collapse of the Soviet Union, 800,000 Russian people ended their life by suicide. The peak came in 1995, with 42 deaths per 100,000 of the population. By 2010 it had fallen dramatically but was still 20 per 100,000. The rate among 15–19-year-olds doubled between 1989 and 2007 to 20 deaths per 100,000 but did not see a fall after that. Other risk behaviours escalated at a similar rate. Numbers of young people addicted to drugs increased 2.7 times, and those suffering from alcoholism sevenfold, while 'the number of recorded HIV cases leapt from around 30,000 in 1994 to more than 250,000 at the end of 1998. Male life expectancy in Russia fell from 64 in 1989 to 58 within four years, with male deaths rising by 60 per cent in the same period.

Why? Hyperinflation, widespread unemployment, falling incomes and the relaxation of restrictions on alcohol availability and use, along with a loss of identity and status for men, and then their difficulties articulating their problems, are widely viewed as causal (Unicef, 1999; Buckland, 2011).

In China, one of the very few countries where the rate of women's suicide was greater than men's, Phillips et al. (2002) found that rural women attempting suicide cited unhappy marriages, spousal abuse, very limited social support structures and easy access to lethal pesticides. A lack of strong religious or legal prohibitions was another feature.

As the example of rural China demonstrates, ready access to lethal means increases risk. Levels of gun ownership in individual American states varies greatly, though overall gun ownership across the country stands at 120.5 per 100 residents. According to the US Centre for Disease Control and Prevention, a total of 24,292 people died from self inflicted gun-related injuries during 2020, more than half of 45,799 recorded suicides (CDC, 2022). The three states with the highest levels of gun ownership also have the highest suicide rate and six of the ten states with the highest levels of gun ownership feature in the ten states with the most suicides. Conversely, Massachusetts and New Jersey have the strictest gun control laws in the US and, along with New York, the lowest suicide rates, less than one third of Montana's 28.9 per 100,000 of the population, the country's worst statistic.

The impulsive use of lethal methods leaves virtually no time for second thoughts or error. Phillips et al. (2002) noted:

> In locations where more lethal methods are frequently used, especially agricultural poisons, there are more deaths among people with a low suicidal intent, some of whom have no mental illness. Our experience in China is that most cases in which the victim has no mental illness are impulsive acts immediately after stressful life events in individuals who have no history of psychological disorders.

The United States has bucked an almost worldwide trend towards a decline in suicide in the 21st century. Its suicide rate has risen by 30 per cent between 2000 and 2020 and now stands at 13.5 per 100,000 of the population, though with a 3 per cent fall between 2019 and 2020. As with Russia decades earlier, 800,000 Americans died during that period (though this is widely recognised as an underestimate because of underreporting of suicide and the deaths also occurred alongside 500,000 deaths from opioid overdoses). We have already looked at the importance of gun ownership and the greater risk associated with impulsive acts in the lack of a presence of mental disorder, but what precipitates a decision to act, whether impulsively or not?

The increase in suicides did not affect the whole of American society. At 23.6 deaths per 100,000, non-Hispanic American Indian or Alaskan Native persons still experience the highest suicide rate in the United States, but these more recent increases have been seen among mostly rural communities, affecting low income White men without a four year college degree. Case and Deaton (2020) linked deaths by suicide with deaths due to alcohol and drug misuse, labelling them 'deaths of despair', causing a *fall* in life expectancy for three consecutive years in America, between 2015–17, for the first time since the Spanish Flu outbreak.[iii] With suicides among non-college educated White men aged 50–54 at twice those of their college educated counterparts, Case and Deaton argue suicide is implacably linked to the collapse of the White working class, and the pathologies that accompany that decline. They cite 'familiar stories about globalisation and automation, changes in social custom that have allowed dysfunctional changes in patterns of marriage and child rearing, the decline in unions, and others', including chronic physical and mental health problems, social isolation, obesity and heavy drinking. With poor access to healthcare, the authors observe that if policy makers 'treat people horribly enough for long enough, bad things happen to them' (Karma, 2020).[iv]

However, an obvious question arises from Case and Deaton's hypothesis. Black and Hispanic populations in the US are often poorer than their White counterparts but less likely to die prematurely through suicide, opioid overdose or alcohol related liver disease.

Reasons are complex. 'Between 2014–19 the suicide rate increased by 30 per cent for Black individuals, from 5.7 to 7.4 100 per 100,000' (Ramchand et al., 2021). However, the group at most significant risk are much younger than the 50–54-year-olds who were the focus of Case and Deaton's work.

It's been postulated that this is the result of a lack of research and, therefore, understanding about the reasons for younger people's suicide. 'Children and teenagers of colour are also less likely to receive mental health care before dying by suicide than White youth' while, in 2019, 20 per cent of White U.S. adults received mental health care, twice that of non-White adults.

So Black people die younger, but nowhere near in the huge numbers of White men aged 50–54 without a college degree. Case and Deaton's work highlights the significance of the losses experienced by this group, not just of employment and money, but status, role, identity, a sense of belongingness. Accompanying this, it's possible a narrative within communities developed in which suicide was an effective response to the pain and distress experienced which became contagious.

Other research suggests the recession that followed the global crash saw 10,000 extra lives lost to suicide in Europe, Canada and the United States between 2007 and 2010. Unemployment, debt and mortgage foreclosure are all seen as contributory factors and unemployed people kill themselves 2.5 times more than those in work (The Economist International, 2018).

Phillips et al. (2002a), in their work on suicides in Chinese women in rural communities, noted the presence of mental disorders in 63 per cent of people completing suicide, significantly lower than in urban, Western communities. What was common to the deceased women, however, were:

- increased negative life events;
- increased and chronic stress in the year before their death;
- decreased quality of life;
- in some cases, the increased impact of the deceased's physical illness on family members;
- increased depressive symptoms in the fortnight before death;
- further increased stress at the time of death;
- previous suicide attempts;
- having relatives, friends or associates with suicidal behaviour.

They conclude that, for the rural women of China, acutely distressed individuals may experience various transient psychological symptoms without meeting the criteria of a mental disorder or personality disorder and that severe stress from acute life events is a more important predictor of suicidal behaviour than the presence of a mental illness.

Looking at suicides in particular, often small, American communities, Abrutyn et al. (2019) found evidence that:

> A series of sudden, shocking, suicide deaths of high-status youth may have triggered the formation of *new locally generalized meanings for suicide that became available, taken-for-granted social facts* [my italics]. The new meanings reinterpreted broadly shared adolescent experiences (exposure to pressure) as a cause of suicide facilitating youth's ability to imagine suicide as something someone *like them* could do to escape.

The authors describe how, for the young people they were studying, a common narrative emerges, in which suicide can seem like a viable option, almost taking on a 'logic' of its own as a means of escape from common problems or experience. Young people experiencing a problem that is perceived as having led their peers to end their life can conclude perhaps this is a way of expressing the distress that adults haven't understood. The contagion effect takes hold within this narrative as death by suicide can seem like an understandable response to a shared problem (Ducharme, 2019).

In the UK, those in the poorest socioeconomic circumstances are approximately ten times more likely to die by suicide than those in the most affluent conditions (Wyllie et al., 2012). The last Adult Psychiatric Morbidity Survey (2014) found those who lived alone or were out of work (either unemployed or economically inactive)[v] were more likely to experience suicidal thoughts, attempt suicide and/or self-harm. Benefit status identified people at particularly high risk. Two-thirds of benefits recipients had suicidal thoughts and 43.2 per cent had made a suicide attempt at some point. A number of studies demonstrated the association between the areas of England most affected by unemployment during the financial crisis and increased suicidal rates. Between 2008 and 2010 there were approximately 800 more suicides among men and 155 more among women than would have been expected based on historical trends (Marsh, 2014).

It's easy to ignore the importance of these broader socioeconomic factors, to think self esteem, motivation and feelings of defeat, of being trapped and hopeless, are linked intrinsically to our internal world whereas there are actually underlying issues far beyond the control of the patient or clinician that exert great influence. And the impact on the individual when their entire community is affected can be devastating.

Equally, there is strong evidence that policy measures can mitigate the effects of recession and economic hardship. Sweden saw no upturn in its rate of suicide after its recession of 1991–92 or the financial crash in 2007, attributed to its healthcare system and government efforts to get people back into work. Japan's success in bringing down unemployment and invigorating its economy saw a decline in suicide rates. Both Mikhael Gorbachev in the 1980s and Vladmir Putin in the early 21st century restricted both alcohol production and sales as part of successful suicide reduction strategies (The Economist International, 2018). The UK's own suicide reduction strategy has contributed to significant reductions in suicide.

The relevance of all this is that, at the time of writing, the UK faces recession amid the highest inflation figures in more than four decades. When adjusted for prices, average earnings excluding bonuses in April 2022 were 3.4 per cent lower than a year earlier, with public sector pay falling by nearly 6 per cent year on year (Atkinson and Aldrick, 2022). 3.7 million people in the UK are in low paid and insecure work, earning less than the real living wage of £10.85 per hour in London and £9.50 outside London.[vi]

More people are economically inactive and energy bills are threatening to force millions into fuel poverty and possible destitution. Trade unions are weaker than they've been in decades (Giupponi and Machin, 2022).

Having narrowed significantly between 1938 and 1979, wealth inequality 'rose considerably' after 1979. Growing wealth inequality in the UK has seen the average income of the richest fifth of the population increase by more than nine per cent between 2012 and 2021, while the average income of the poorest fifth of the population has stayed the same over those nine years (McRae and Westwater, 2022; The Equality Trust, 2022).

Of note, while wealth inequality, low pay and job insecurity all disproportionately affect Black and ethnic minority people, UK suicide rates, only recently analysed for ethnicity, show that for females mixed/multiple ethnic groups had the highest rate of suicide, with the rate for White men equalling that for males from mixed/multiple ethnic groups (see Figure 1.3).

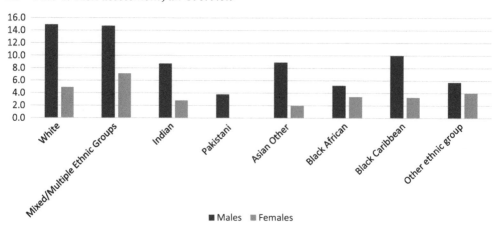

Figure 1.3 Age standardised rates of death per 100,000 from suicide by ethnic group in England and Wales, 2017–2019

Source: APMS 2014, NHS Digital. *Copyright © 2016, Health and Social Care Information Centre*

These levels of social and economic instability in our communities, affecting our families as well as us as individuals, matter profoundly. Noted sociologist Émile Durkheim highlighted more than a century ago that despair and then suicide result when people's material and social circumstances fall below their expectations (Gawande, 2020).

If history does repeat itself, there will likely be a significant increase in people experiencing suicidal ideation, harming themselves and even ending their lives. In these circumstances healthcare leaders and organisations need to be pressing for economic policies that support the most vulnerable, with services that are geared up to meet increased demand as well as ensuring their clinical staff are as knowledgeable and skilled in risk assessment and management as possible.

Suicide: a statistical overview[vii]

If each suicide is an individual tragedy, statistics about suicide are obviously useful in identifying trends, demographic variations and risk factors etc. However, they must be treated with a degree of caution. For example, there are differences in how some countries arrive at a verdict of suicide, complicating international comparisons. As noted below, a new legal standard has been introduced, allowing coroners to reach a conclusion about suicide rather than verdict, which will almost certainly alter the numbers identified and reflect more realistically actual deaths – it has long been asserted that the numbers of suicides in the UK are underestimated by at least thirty per cent and as much as fifty per cent for young people (Gil, 2017).

The Adult Psychiatric Morbidity Survey (McManus et al., 2016), having surveyed 7,500 people, provides significant evidence about people's experience of suicidal thoughts and how that translates into suicide attempts. Their research estimates:

- 1 in 5 (20 per cent) people in England (approximately 11.3 million adults) have suicidal thoughts;
- 1 in 15 (6.6 per cent) people in England (approximately 3.7 million adults) attempt suicide;

Table 1.4 Lifetime suicidal thoughts and suicide attempts by age and sex

All adults				Age				
	16–24 per cent	25–34 per cent	35–44 per cent	45–54 per cent	55–64 per cent	65–74 per cent	75 + per cent	All per cent
Men								
Suicidal thoughts	19.3	21.1	21.1	20.7	22.5	11.9	7.1	18.7
Suicidal attempts	5.4	8.0	6.5	5.4	5.4	3.5	1.0	5.4
Women								
Suicidal thoughts	34.6	24.1	22.8	26.6	22.9	11.7	8.8	22.4
Suicidal attempts	12.7	9.1	9.5	8.2	8.6	3.7	2.1	8.0
All adults								
Suicidal thoughts	26.8	22.6	21.9	23.7	22.7	11.8	8.1	20.6
Suicidal attempts	9.0	8.5	8.0	6.8	7.0	3.6	1.7	6.7

Source: APMS 2014, NHS Digital. Copyright © 2016, Health and Social Care Information Centre

- 46 per cent of people who die by suicide had a known mental health condition;
- more than 1 in 3 people who die from suicide are under the influence of alcohol at the time of death.

McManus et al. (2016) discovered suicidal thoughts and suicide attempts were most common among White British communities (see Figure 1.4). More women (22.4 per cent) than men (18.7 per cent) have thoughts of taking their own life at some point, and it's more common in people of working-age than those aged 65 or older.

Though women experience suicidal thoughts more frequently than men, there are significant differences occurring in ethnic groups. The 'Mixed, Multiple and Other' ethnic group demonstrate this, with more than twice as many women affected (see Figure 1.4). Unsurprisingly, this group then experience the highest number of suicide attempts among women. 'White Other' men are most affected by suicidal thoughts but more 'Black/Black British' men go on to attempt suicide than those from other ethnic groups, though it's men with a 'White British' and 'Mixed/Multiple Ethnic Origin' who go on to complete suicide the most. Almost 35 per cent of women aged 16–24 have suicidal thoughts and nearly 13 per cent of women in this age group attempted to end their life, more than double that of men. They also have high levels of self-harm and wider psychiatric morbidity (McManus et al., 2016; ONS, 2020).[viii, ix]

Both suicidal thoughts and suicide attempts were higher among women, the one exception being men aged 65–74, who experience marginally more suicidal thoughts than women in the same range (see Table 1.4).

The precipitating life events for women who attempt suicide tend to be losses or crises in significant social or family relationships. As with men, suicide is more common among women who are single or recently separated, divorced or widowed. However, women are more likely than men to have stronger social supports, to feel their relationships are deterrents to suicide, and seek psychiatric and other medical intervention (Cooper et al., 2005; Murphy 1998).

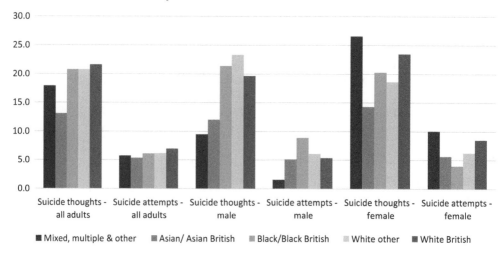

Figure 1.4 Lifetime suicidal thoughts and suicide attempts (age-standardised), by ethnic group and sex

Source: APMS 2014, NHS Digital. Copyright © 2016, Health and Social Care Information Centre

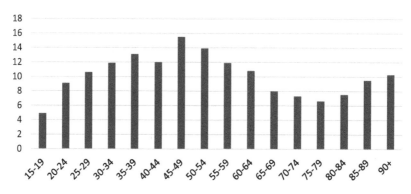

Figure 1.5 Age-specific suicide rates per 100,000, all adults: by five-year age group, England and Wales, 2020 (Baker, 2021)

In terms of historic trends, male suicide peaked in 1905 and 1935 at 20.3 per 100,000 and female suicide peaked in 1960. Apart from a reverse in 1980, female suicide has steadily declined since. The trend for men during the same period is different. For men, 20 years of decline were followed by a sustained increase between 1970 and 1990, by which time it had almost returned to its 1950 level. The 1990s and early 21st century saw the numbers falling again before fluctuating increases since 2008. The overall fall in numbers is largely due to an almost 50 per cent drop in female suicides between 1981 and 2020. The fall in male suicides in the same period was only 20 per cent (Baker, 2021).

The highest suicide rates fall between the ages of 35 and 54 in both men and women, the increase is much sharper among women than men (see Figure 1.5). There was also a largely unexplained drop from 18.9 to 9.5 per 100,000 in all adults aged over 50.

Although the drop in male suicides during this 40-year period was only 20 per cent, the number of men aged over 50 in England and Wales ending their life effectively halved (see Figure 1.6). The only significant change in the under-50s was seen in the 40–44 age group, which had a fall from 15.6 to 12.0 (Baker, 2021).

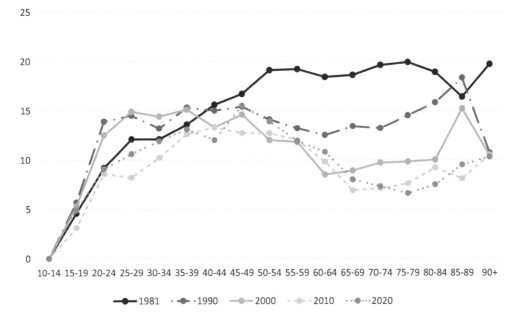

Figure 1.6 Age-specific suicide rates: by five-year age group, England and Wales, 1981 to 2020 (Baker 2021)

The difference in rates of suicide across the UK and Northern Ireland has been stable since 2015, with Scotland consistently having the highest rate (see Figure 1.7).

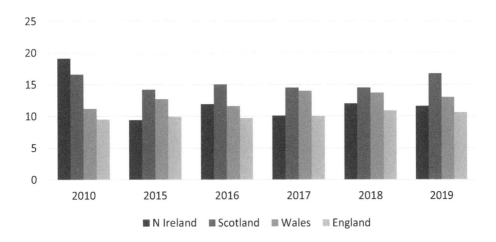

Figure 1.7 Suicide rates per 100,000 population by year of death, by UK country

Suicide in other numbers

- 75 per cent of all suicide deaths are male. While male deaths from suicide are greater in all age groups, the ratio varies in different age ranges.
- The suicide rate equates to approximately 1 per cent of UK deaths.
- Approximately 25 per cent of people completing suicide had been in recent contact with mental health services.
- Over one-fifth of individuals dying by suicide have not been adherent to medication in the preceding month and nearly one-third have disengaged from services.
- 160–200 psychiatric inpatients die by suicide annually, most commonly by hanging; this figure has fallen during the past decade.
- The period of highest risk after discharge from in-patient care is the first 7 days, with most suicides occurring on day three post discharge.

When looked at in terms of deprivation in England, suicide reflects exactly the country's socioeconomic structure, with suicides between 2017–19 in the most deprived 10 per cent of areas at 14.1 per 100,000, almost double that of the rate in the least deprived areas (Baker, 2022).

However, looking at broad occupational groups at most risk of suicide in 2020 (see Figure 1.8), it's skilled tradesmen – almost exclusively made up of males. However, broken down into more specific areas of male occupation, the highest ranking are 'elementary construction occupations', followed by 'construction and building trades' and factory workers. Among women by far the highest suicide rate is among 'care workers and home carers', almost double that of the next highest, 'sales and retail assistants'. Nurses rate the fifth highest.

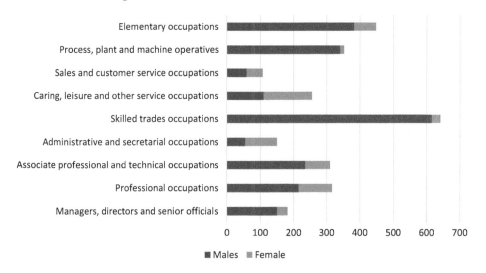

Figure 1.8 Number of suicides for major group occupations, males and females aged between 20 to 64 years in 2020

Source: Suicide by Occupation in England: 2011 to 2020. www.ons.gov.uk

However, the question that lies behind all these statistics is why? This is a question that can be looked at in two ways. Is there a range of factors that combine to take an individual down the pathway to suicide? The other is the wider context.

O'Connor and Kirtley (2018) attempt to answer the first question with their Integrated Motivational – Volitional Model of Suicidal Behaviour.[x] It doesn't ignore the social and environmental context of suicide risk but links this with early life adversity or trauma as an unequivocal suicide risk factor, in turn linking these with 'epigenetic changes in genes, the dysregulation of cortisol, [and] difficulties with attachment and relationships', stating 'the overarching premise of the IMV model is that the pre-motivational factors have their effect on suicide risk through their influence on the constructs within the motivational and volitional phases'.

There are three stages to the model. First, they describe the pre-motivational phase, constituting background factors and triggering events. This is made up of a combination of:

- a predisposition or biological, cognitive and genetic vulnerability for developing a pathological state (diathesis), e.g. decreased serotonergic neurotransmission;
- factors such as early life adversity, including trauma, a high level of perfectionism and high levels of self criticism, with the person believing significant others have high expectations of them. This can lead to feelings of 'defeat' when not attained or the person experiences an interpersonal crisis they can't resolve;
- rapid societal changes, socio-economic deprivation and inequality.

Already predisposed, the person then experiences a 'triggering' event, e.g. a relationship breakup or crisis, significant loss etc.

Second is the motivational phase, when the formation of suicidal ideation and intentions occurs. The individual experiences a sense of 'entrapment' which can be internal, triggered by painful thoughts and feelings, or external, triggered by a desire to escape from events or experiences in the outside world. In both cases it results from feelings of defeat and/or humiliation, often when the person perceives they have failed to reach a particular goal or experienced social rejection and loss. Perceiving no way of escaping either those feelings or the situation, the person is likely to feel agitated and ruminate in a way that is brooding rather than reflective. This can then lead to hopelessness, or a pervasive sense of pessimism for the future, with thoughts of suicide as 'a way out'.

The person is also likely to be experiencing difficulty in social problem solving and autobiographical memory biases, or difficulty accessing memories of positive experiences with a bias towards either remembering everything negative or even reframing positive experiences as negative.

So called 'motivational moderators' that once would have been protective, including factors allowing the individual to see positive, less painful alternatives, the ability to adapt their goals, as well as a sense of belonging and connectedness, become absent. The person is left feeling isolated and disconnected, with little or no social support, thinking they're a burden on others. Coupled with depleted resilience and less negative attitudes towards suicide, this increases the likelihood that the sense of entrapment will convert suicidal ideation into suicidal intent as the person perceives they are alone, don't matter, and neither they nor anyone else can find a solution to a situation that is unbearable.

Their third phase concerns volition, when suicidal thoughts and impulses transition to suicidal behaviour. 'Volitional moderators' are vital for transition from suicidal ideation to suicidal intent. It's their presence that increases the likelihood of a suicide attempt. The acquired capability for suicide, or the person losing their fear of death and increasing their physical pain tolerance are volitional moderators while having access to a means of suicide that the person would use is an environmental volitional moderator. Social volitional moderators include exposure to the suicidal behaviour of others known to the person, e.g. a family member or a friend.

While impulsivity is another key factor, planning makes death more likely. The two aren't mutually exclusive, as the person may have developed a plan but then act upon it impulsively. Imagining, or fantasising, about their death and even what will happen afterwards is another significant factor in advancing the act itself.

When looking at those broader factors, it's still necessary to consider why people end their life when they're unemployed or suffering because of government policies of austerity. What is it about being between the ages of 45 and 49? Is there something specific that occurs to young women between the ages of 16 and 24 that a quarter of them self-harm and almost as many have suicidal thoughts?

Barnes et al. (2016) set about investigating these questions, particularly referencing economic hardship in a time of recession and austerity. Their conclusion, after in depth interviews with 19 people who had attended hospital following an episode of self-harm in which economic hardship or the impact of austerity had contributed, was that, 'in many cases problems accumulated and felt unresolvable'. For others, the self-harm was triggered by a specific event such as a call from a debt collector or change in benefits. Other factors were present, including 'abuse, neglect, bullying, domestic violence, mental health problems, relationship difficulties, bereavements and low esteem'. The people interviewed experienced a sense of despair and worthlessness, which was exacerbated and increased their vulnerability to self-harm.

There is a degree of correlation between the numbers of male suicides by age and the numbers of men whose marriages end in divorce. For example, in 2016 (the most recent year for which divorce statistics are available), the age group among males with the highest suicide rate is 40–44 at 24.1 per 100,000, with those aged 45–49 ending their life at a rate of 23.1 per 100,000. That year the divorce rate for men peaked at 13.8 per 100,000 for those aged 45–49 and 13.6 in the 40–44 age group.

What is clear is that these external events on their own do not precipitate suicide but play an important part in affecting the person. These themes can be understood through the cry of pain and emotional cascade models and will be explored in more depth when we look at clinical risk indicators and the suicidal crossroads (see page 39), as well as how they fit with models of self-harm and suicide (see page 23). What is crucial, clinically, is how we understand how the individual integrates these experiences, what they think, how they feel, how they perceive them. As we shall see, there are ways in which these things can be explored directly in an assessment.

When thinking about suicide, we should always remember that behind these statistics lies untold and unique personal tragedies. Not just for the person who died but for loved ones, families, friends, colleagues and even those healthcare professionals who have tried to help the person remain safe. If any death by suicide can be avoided, it is a victory for hope and the belief things can be better.

So perhaps the last word in this section should go not to an academic or clinician but a writer, whose close friend, the author and poet Sylvia Plath, ended her life aged 30. 'Suicide is a closed world, with its own irresistible logic', wrote A. Alvarez in *The Savage God*, a response to Sylvia's death. 'Everything makes sense and follows its own strict rules; yet, at the same time, everything is also different, perverted, upside down'.

The Coronavirus pandemic

Analysis by the ONS looked at the period of April–July 2020, which overlapped with the first national lockdown. The data showed a fall in suicides across England and Wales for that period from recent years and 9.2 per 100,000 compared to 11.3 for the same period in 2019, largely due to a fall in male suicide (Baker, 2021).

However, that is not the whole story. Large scale surveys by MIND (2021) and the Mental Health Foundation (Kousoulis et al., 2022) have tracked the impact of the pandemic, lockdowns and the socioeconomic disruption to people's lives. Both found people of all ages and from all strata of society experiencing long term mental distress but that this was more profound for vulnerable groups, including those with pre-existing mental health problems and young people. An increase in suicidal thoughts was picked up by the research commissioned by The Mental Health Foundation. By November 2021, 12 per cent of those questioned, down from 14 per cent in September, were experiencing suicidal thoughts but 33 per cent of those with a pre-existing mental health problems were affected and 34 per cent of people were aged 18–24.

Suicide and specific groups[xi]

Suicide and young people

Suicide accounts for almost 23 per cent of all deaths of people aged 15–24, and is the second most common cause of death in young people after accidental death (Office for National Statistics, 20017). Other important statistics about young people and suicide are:

- suicides by people under 18 increased from 85 in 2009 to 98 in 2016 before a sharp, unaccounted for increase in 2017, when it rose to 135. Following that there was a fall back to 108 by 2019;
- unique in all age groups, 49 per cent of young patients who died by suicide were female;
- the period 2009–19 also saw an increase in deaths by girls aged 16 and boys aged 17, and by a rise in deaths by hanging/strangulation in the under 18s, for whom it is the most commonly used method;
- 19 per cent were under the care of a mental health team in the 12 months prior to their death;11 per cent were from a minority ethnic group;
- 74 per cent had a history of self-harm;
- 25 per cent had used the internet to research suicide, visited websites encouraging suicide or signaled their intent.

Suicide and substance misuse

Substance misuse has long been recognised as a risk factor for suicide and suicide attempts. Alcohol and drugs affect thinking and reasoning ability and can act as depressants. They can decrease inhibitions, making impulsive actions of a dangerous nature more likely and increase the likelihood of a depressed person making a suicide attempt. Alcohol and drugs are thought to be of particular significance in suicides that appear to be impulsive and are particularly implicated in the suicides of young men.

As many as 70 per cent of men and 40 per cent of women who attempt suicide have blood alcohol concentrations exceeding the legal limit. The risk persists even after abstinence has been established. Although an estimated 40 per cent of all alcoholics attempt suicide at least once, it is estimated that up to 25 per cent of people formerly addicted to alcohol will end their life by suicide after having found sobriety (www.addictions.uk).

Other statistics highlight the scale of the problem:

- estimates suggest that about 15 per cent of people who misuse alcohol may eventually kill themselves;
- men are nine times more likely than women to misuse alcohol. Men diagnosed with alcohol addiction are six times as likely to die by suicide as men in the general population;
- although women are less likely than men to misuse alcohol, those who do are at a much greater risk of suicide than men, with a suicide rate twenty times that of the general population (Harris and Barraclough, 1997).

Establishing whether or not drug related deaths are suicides is far more complicated. However, it is worth noting that there were 4561 deaths related to drug poisoning in England and Wales in 2020, a 3.8 per cent increase from the previous year. The ratio of male to female deaths is different from suicide, in that women account for 32 per cent of those deaths. For males, the death rate is highest in the 45–49 age group, or people born in the 1970s, while the North East of England has the highest death rate from drug misuse. Almost half of all drug related deaths involve opiates (ONS, 2021). There were 1321 suspected drug related deaths in Scotland in 2020, a huge increase from the 527 deaths in 2013. The most at risk group were 35–44 year olds and more than two thirds were male (National Records of Scotland, 2022).

Suicide and mental illness

In a study of 6367 cases of suicide by current or recent mental health patients between April 2000 and December 2004 (Appleby et al., 2006), the primary diagnosis of known patients at time of death was:

1. affective disorder (present in 2821 or 46 per cent of cases);
2. schizophrenia and other delusional disorders (present in 1145 or 19 per cent of cases);
3. drug and alcohol dependence (present in 206 or 11 per cent of cases);
4. personality disorder (present in 518 or 8 per cent of cases).

Mental health patients[xii]

Between 2009–2019, 5218 patients (29 per cent) who died by suicide were in acute care settings (in-patients, under crisis resolution/home treatment), or had been recently discharged from in-patient care. This is an average of 1661 suicides per year during this period. Deaths by hanging/strangulation among this group rose, especially in female patients and in patients aged under 25. The number of deaths by self-poisoning also increased (Appleby et al., 2022).

Most patients who died had previously self-harmed (64 per cent) and there were high proportions of those with alcohol and drug misuse – 47 per cent and 37 per cent respectively.

5218 (29 per cent) patient deaths during this period occurred while the person was in an acute care setting, including inpatients (6 per cent), post discharge care (15 per cent) and crisis resolution/home treatment (14 per cent). Nonetheless, this represents a fall over this period, from 92.8 per 100,000 mental health service users in 2009 to 47.8 per 100,000 in 2019. The ratio of men to women remains broadly the same as that of the general population, i.e. 3:1.

Almost half (46 per cent) of those who died had been in contact with mental health services in the week before death. Significantly, 84 per cent were viewed by clinicians as at low or no short-term risk – a figure that has not much changed in the past two decades. Of those who went on to die, 24 per cent had missed their last appointment with services and 13 per cent were non-adherent with medication. Although inpatient deaths fell from 95 in 2009 to 67 in 2019, 56 per cent of those who died as inpatients in 2019 had left the ward with the agreement of staff (Appleby et al., 2022).

Inpatients are most vulnerable in the first week after admission. The highest risk was in the first 1–2 weeks after discharge and the highest number of deaths occurred on day 3 post discharge.

Between the years 2009 and 2019, major risk factors for patients are:

* marital status – 73 per cent are unmarried;
* gender – 66 per cent are male;
* living alone – 48 per cent live alone;
* employment status – 39 per cent are unemployed;
* age – 13 per cent are 65 and over.

Anniversaries remain a potential trigger. Between 2011 and 2019, an average of 109 people ended their life on or near an anniversary or significant date.

41 per cent of patients dying by suicide had been diagnosed with an affective disorder, i.e. depression or bipolar affective disorder.

Methods of suicide

The method by which an individual chooses to end their life is influenced by wider events in society. For example, in the 19th century the introduction of domestic gas was quickly taken up as a means for ending one's life and was the most common means of suicide for men in the 1950s and 1960s. The increase in gassing deaths between the wars was not matched by a decline in other methods of suicide and overall numbers rose. Although hanging was the most common method of suicide for men in the 1860s, the following century saw a decline before it rose to become the most common means from the 1960s to the present day. For women, hanging was the second most common method throughout the nineteenth century before declining. It increased again in the 1960s and again after 1996, and since then it has become the most common method of suicide, supplanting self poisoning.

The change to natural gas – which is not poisonous – led to a dramatic fall in poisoning for men and women. Men turned to self poisoning through car exhaust fumes but reductions in the levels of carbon monoxide in petrol saw a steep decline in that as a method (Thomas and Gunnell, 2010).

Hanging and strangulation rose by more than 1,000 per year between 2010 and 2019, when it peaked at 3,861. Self poisoning has remained steady at just over 1,015–1,408 over the last decade. Jumping/multiple injuries is next most common but peaked at 646 in 2014 and has steadily declined to 502 in 2019.

One study of people who survived attempted hanging revealed:

> Hanging was adopted or contemplated for two main reasons: the anticipated nature of a death from hanging; and accessibility. Those favouring hanging anticipated a certain, rapid and painless death with little awareness of dying and believed it was a "clean" method that would not damage the body or leave harrowing images for others. Materials for hanging were easily accessed and respondents considered it "simple" to perform without the need for planning or technical knowledge.
>
> (Biddle et al., 2010)

In 2019 Northern Ireland (58 per cent) and Wales (54 per cent) had a higher proportion of suicide by hanging/strangulation compared to the UK average (46 per cent).

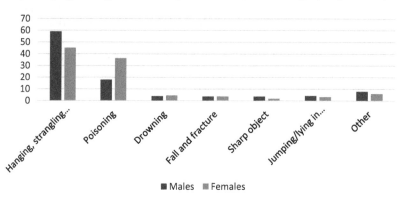

Figure 1.9 Proportion of suicide by method and sex, 2018
Source: ONS (2019)

At assessment and presenting symptoms at last contact

In one study of 6,36 cases of suicide by current or recent mental health patients (Appleby et al., 2006), the following symptoms were noted to have been present at the last clinical contact before death:

1. emotional distress (present in 1,971 cases);
2. depressive illness (present in 1,706 cases);
3. hopelessness (present in 841 cases);
4. suicidal ideas (present in 780 cases);
5. recent self-harm (present in 770 cases);
6. increased use of alcohol (present in 697 cases);
7. deterioration in physical health (present in 463 cases);
8. delusions or hallucinations (present in 427 cases).

The new civil standard for defining suicide and possible numbers of actual deaths through suicide

In May 2019 the Court of Appeal in England and Wales handed down a ruling on the determination of suicide at inquests that is likely to affect the national suicide rate and influence policy priorities. That ruling upheld a 2018 decision taken in the High Court, which had determined a conclusion based 'on the balance of probabilities' about whether or not someone had ended their life by suicide should be the civil standard of proof required. Previously, a verdict had been required, meeting the criminal standard, which was 'beyond reasonable doubt'. The lowering of this threshold is expected to lead to an increase in deaths recorded as suicide (Appleby et al., 2019).

Clinical risk indicators for suicide

Clinical risk indicators for suicide are factors identified in people who have either ended their life or attempted to do so. They are derived from large scale population studies and can be used by the assessor to identify key issues that *may* highlight areas of risk in the individual's background. However, this does not necessarily indicate, for instance, that someone of male gender in their early fifties, recently unemployed and depressed is going to kill himself. Nor does it indicate that someone without these factors in his presentation apart from current suicidal thoughts and intent should not be considered likely to kill himself. Identification of the risk factors highlighted here should occur during a comprehensive assessment and be judged in the context of the individual's overall presentation.

Nevertheless, the number of known risk factors present in any individual's personal circumstances must be taken into account in that person's risk management.

Table 1.5 Clinical risk indicators for suicide (adapted from Morgan, 2000)

Historical	Cognitive
Previous self-harm	Current suicidal thoughts/ideation
Family history of suicide	Severe psychic anxiety
Previous use of violent methods	Suicide plan
Physical	Belief of no control over self/events
Chronic physical illness	Ruminations
Chronic physical pain	**Behaviour**
Emotions	Disengaged from services
Hopelessness	Poor adherence to psychiatric treatment
Helplessness	Access/willingness to use lethal means
Diagnosis	**Social**
Depression	Unemployed/retired
Psychosis	Separated/widowed/divorced
Alcohol and/or drug misuse	Family concerned about risk
Post natal depression	Lack of social support
Puerperal psychosis	**Other**
Verbal	Male gender
Expressed intent	Discharged from psychiatric hospital within last 3 days to 2 weeks

The suicidal crossroads?

Suicidal behaviour seems to increase when these factors converge:

1. precipitating stressors occur in the recent **past,** e.g. the break up of a relationship, bereavement, loss of job etc;

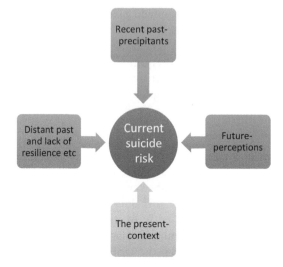

Figure 1.10 Factors affecting current suicide risk

2. these stressors resonate with **more distant** stressors or traits that have hindered the development of the person's coping strategies and resilience as well as a 'rewriting' of the person's history that blots out most positive achievements and events;
3. the context of the **present** difficulties, e.g. ruminating about what is perceived to be happening and experiencing the situation as unbearable, feeling hopeless and:
4. greater hopelessness is a function of perceptions of the **future** which are lacking positivity, rather than filled with ideas of a negative future (Williams et al., 2005), with the individual:

   a. literally unable to see positive outcomes and;
   b. feeling trapped and unable to identify solutions to the problems they face (see Figure 4).

Feelings of hopelessness are highly correlated with suicide risk and it should be remembered that this is not always associated with depression. There are specific assessment scales that focus on hopelessness that can be useful but it is important to explore the extent and impact of this on the person's suicidal ideation.

Possible protective factors

Wherever possible, involving the person in identifying what might help them, what has reduced the risk before and why, is an essential part of any assessment and one that is often neglected. Part of this process is an examination of what individual protective factors might affect any potential risk(s). These will be unique to the individual and may be long standing. Trying to understand them and their function is important in your assessment of risk and gaining a greater understanding of the person you're conversing with. Equally, you should explore what may impact upon them. For example, someone with strong religious beliefs that have acted as a powerful deterrent to attempting suicide may be at serious risk if they experience a crisis of faith. Similarly, the loss of a relationship that has previously been very supportive and been a safeguard against suicidal feelings is likely to increase the risk. Part of the assessment is to explore how longstanding these factors are, how strong they are and why they have been protective. Tools such as the Structured Assessment of Protective Factors (De Vogel et al., 2012) can be used not only to help with this element of the assessment but also to balance the assessment of risk and provide a more accurate judgement of any risk.

It's also essential not to make assumptions. For example, children and family members might be viewed as strong and positive protective factors by the clinician assessing the patient. But the patient may have concluded, however mistakenly, that they are a burden on their family, and their children and family would be better off without them. It may simply be that friction within the family or with children is a particular stressor and being apart is the protective factor.

Possible protective factors may include:

- personal resilience;
- good problem solving skills;
- future plans/hope for the future;
- strong religious faith or spiritual belief;
- belief that suicide is wrong;
- family responsibilities, e.g. as carer;
- a strong relationship with spouse/partner;
- strong social support;
- relationships and integration within community;
- economic security in older age;
- early identification and appropriate treatment of mental health problems;
- fear of pain and/or self-harm (O'Brien and Hart 2013).

From this, an element of the risk management plan emerges. It is to support any known protective factors and, if any have been weakened by events or circumstance, to try and help the person rebuild them.

Assessing the risk of self-harm or suicide for people with emotionally unstable personality disorder/borderline personality disorder

Depression is the mental disorder that carries the greatest risk of suicide. This is reflected in much of the material in the *Pocket Guide* and, particularly, the thinking and emotional responses that appear to accompany suicidal acts. However, assessing risk in people diagnosed with emotionally unstable personality disorder often seems to prove most challenging for clinicians and clinical teams. Possible reasons for this are numerous and cannot be discussed in detail here. Nor can the diagnosis and disorder itself. The focus of this section is only on the principles of addressing risk(s) related to how the disorder affects the person experiencing it. Although these principles are largely the same as they would be for anyone else, it is nonetheless worth exploring some of the issues that arise. Some have their origins in the nature of the disorder itself but others can be directly linked to the structure and organisation of mental health services and the functioning of teams.

The term 'emotionally unstable disorder' only came into usage relatively recently but attempts to describe and understand the experience of people exhibiting what might be termed intense and often very different emotions within a short space of time. This phenomena can be found as far back as in ancient Greek literature. Doctors and writers in the 19th century described people experiencing emotional instability and erratic patterns of behaviour and the term 'borderline' related to 'insanity' was coined in the latter part of the 1800s. The term 'borderline personality disorder' (BPD) evolved from Adolph Stern's 1938 description of a group of patients he'd been seeing who seemed to live on the borderline between neurosis and psychosis. Others thought it stood on the borderline of a range of disorders, often leading to misdiagnosis and inappropriate treatment. It was not classified into a formal diagnosis until 1980 when is appeared in the DSM-III. This was slightly revised for the DSM-IV and then retained, unchanged, in the latest version (Biskin and Paris, 2012), despite criticism that the term 'borderline' doesn't adequately describe the person's experience of the disorder. The International Classification of Disease of the World Health Organisation (ICD-10) now uses the term emotionally unstable personality disorder or EUPD (F60.3) as a primary diagnosis, with two sub types: impulsive and borderline, though there are suggestions that it should be renamed complex post traumatic stress disorder, highlighting its relationship to childhood trauma and stress responses and because both EUPD and BPD are thought to be stigmatising.

However, many people will have been diagnosed with the disorder without having gone through a formal assessment and the structured and semi structured interviews required to formalise the diagnosis. Moreover, many clinicians will use the term 'PD' as a generalised reference to personality disorder without being absolutely sure of the specific criteria for different types of personality disorder, including emotionally unstable personality disorder and borderline personality disorder. There is no doubt that the term PD is, in itself, sometimes used in a pejorative and derogatory way by clinicians when being used to describe patients.

A person must meet at least five of the nine criteria from the DSM-5 to be diagnosed (American Psychiatric Association, 2013). This means 256 different combinations can lead to a diagnosis (Biskin and Paris, 2012). The diagnostic criteria are:

1. Frantic efforts to avoid real or imagined abandonment.
2. Unstable and intense interpersonal relationships – alternating between idealisation and devaluation.
3. Identity disturbance – unstable sense of self.
4. Impulsivity.
5. Recurrent suicidal behaviour, threats, gestures or self-harming.
6. Affective instability inc. anxiety.
7. Feelings of emptiness, worthlessness.
8. Inappropriate anger.
9. Transient, stress related paranoid ideation or severe dissociative symptoms.

The lifetime prevalence is approximately 5.9 per cent and point prevalence (the prevalence measured at a particular point in time) 1.6 per cent. However, almost 10 per cent of outpatients and 20 per cent of inpatients will have been diagnosed with the disorder.

Controversially, a predominance of women is diagnosed with the disorder – as many as 75–80 per cent in some studies. Critics argue this is evidence of a gendered diagnosis. Shaw and Procter (2004) write 'throughout history, society has created multiple categories for women who do not fit into society's norms and expectations' and 'women already marginalised by society are further stigmatised by BPD. [It] has always been a diagnosis of exclusion from mainstream mental health services, women are marginalised and stigmatised ... by descriptions such as manipulative, attention-seeking nuisances'.

Critics of the diagnosis also highlight the subjective nature of the criteria. What, for instance, is 'inappropriate anger'? When does a relationship become unstable or intense and is that a psychiatric problem? In a sharp rebuke to mental health clinicians, a critical theorist and activist collective, Recovery in the Bin, issued a 36-point 'Simple Guide to Avoid Receiving a Diagnosis of Personality Disorder', including:

- 'Try not to be female'.
- 'You cannot be seen to like some staff members more than others (this is SPLITTING behaviour)'.
- 'Do not make statements, which can be interpreted as black and white thinking. For example, the nurses all hate me. Try instead to make unrealistic, robot-like, rational statements such as 'Enid, Mary, Silvia, John, Mark and Boteng have all shown epic disdain at my presence on the ward, but an agency nurse once smiled at me in 1992'.
- 'Never phone the crisis team and say you'd like another visit (tick box dependency issues)' (Recovery In The Bin, 2016).

However, the high ratio of women diagnosed may also be explained by the way men respond differently to the disorder. Biskin and Paris (2012) note that 'men and women with similar psychological problems may express distress differently' and that men may not seek treatment but use illicit substances and alcohol more. They may also commit crimes that either lead to them being imprisoned and/or labelled as 'anti social'. Studies have also shown that as many as 30 per cent of people completing suicide were men diagnosed with borderline personality disorder post mortem (through interviews with family members), with very few ever having been treated.

The disorder's causes are complex, nor fully understood, but there is a growing consensus that brain development is affected by an interaction between genetic, neurobiological and psychosocial influences. Neurobiological research and neuroimaging studies have shown differences in crucial areas of the brain, including the hippocampus, amygdala, prefrontal cortex and hypothalamic pituitary adrenal axis. These are attributed with problems with memory, creating a greater sense of ongoing threat and consequent anxiety, more intense and prolonged emotions, creating stronger memories of stressful events and people being less functional in their decision making in response to these heightened emotions, with excessive stress hormones being produced that then undermine coping skills and resilience, which in turn create more intense stressful reactions (Kulacaoglu and Kose, 2018).

The most significant risk factor for EUPD/BPD, however, is childhood trauma, though the relationship is not entirely clear, as not every sufferer of the disorder will describe childhood trauma and not everyone experiencing childhood trauma develops the disorder. Trauma can take the form of, among other things, sexual, physical or psychological abuse; early parental loss or separation; parents abusing alcohol and/or drugs and some mental disorders, including a major depressive disorder and PTSD. While Kulacaoglu and Kose (2018) state 'sexual abuse history is not found as a risk factor for BPD', Klaus Leib et al. (2004) note that 'childhood sexual abuse … is reported by 40–71 per cent of inpatients with borderline personality disorder'.

Common features are:

- dichotomous thinking (often referred to as 'black and white' thinking), extreme views that represent the opposite of each other and which seem impossible to reconcile;
- difficulty maintaining relationships;

- rapidly changing – often extreme – emotions, with impulsive reactions to what is happening around them;
- impulsivity;
- it's also possible, if the person does have a history of abuse or neglect from significant people in their lives, e.g. parents, family members, carers, that they will have difficulty trusting others, something which the clinician will have to take into account in developing and maintaining a therapeutic relationship. This can be even more challenging in a risk assessment, especially if the patient's experiences of mental health services and emergency departments has been variable.

These all carry risk to the person and, occasionally, others, including neglect of their physical and mental health, substance misuse and impulsive, dangerous acts such as promiscuity and unprotected sex, risky driving and overspending. They are also the source of a lot of distress, with extreme feelings of emptiness, sadness, numbness and a lack of certainty about their identity or what they want from life. They may experience problems with attention, cognitive flexibility, planning, learning and memory.

The behaviour of people with the disorder can often be perceived as challenging; they are often labelled as 'manipulative' and/or 'attention seeking' and may even be described as the person who is 'splitting' the team. These misunderstandings about people suffering with this disorder only add to the stigma associated with it. Manipulation requires both skill and subtlety. As Marsha Linehan (2009) points out, the problematic behaviours of BPD are anything but subtle and skilful. In a piece for *The New York Times*, where she answers questions from readers, she responds to a woman desperate to help her parents cope with 'manipulation' in the form of her sister's non-lethal self-harm and suicide threats:

> It is true that people — including therapists — who spend time around people with borderline personality disorder often feel manipulated and feel like they are held hostage. Behaviours such as suicide threats often have that effect on people. It is really a tragedy for both parties when that happens.

> It is rare, however, that a person with borderline personality disorder is actually trying to "manipulate," that is, to manage, control or influence in a subtle, devious, or underhand manner (Oxford dictionary); or to handle with mental or intellectual skill (also from the Oxford dictionary). A suicide threat or attempt is certainly not subtle or devious. It is right out in the open!

Elsewhere, Linehan (2015) describes these behaviours as typically desperate, unskilful attempts to have one's emotional needs met and talks about symptoms of BPD as deficits in the skills of emotion regulation, distress tolerance and interpersonal effectiveness that most people without the disorder might take for granted.

'Attention seeking behaviour' can be reframed and viewed as seeking validation, approval, praise, admiration, care and even love. This requires self awareness in knowing what type of attention we want and why, the social skills to achieve that goal, resilience and adaptability to try something different if the first attempt isn't successful and to marry external validation with internal self acceptance or self validation, a sense of self worth that does not require any external input. The ways in which we seek the attention of others are learned from infancy through a dynamic process of exhibiting behaviours that garner the desired response and then repeating them consistently. These require consistent responses from parents, care givers etc. Looking at the early years' experience of people with BPD, with the resulting dichotomous thinking, difficult relationships and emotional instability, it is clear they are going to struggle to both develop and then use the skills required to seek attention in healthy and adaptive ways, particularly when stressed, feeling threatened or anxious.

Perhaps the most troubling misperception is that patients with BPD/EUPD can 'split' teams, as if the person is able to consciously influence the minds of large numbers of people in the staff team. In this context, the term 'splitting' takes on an accusatory nature. There are numerous accounts of opposing views about a patient being held within a clinical team. The first known written description of this was Tom Main's 'The Ailment' (1957). In these instances, staff experience complex and intense emotions in relation to a patient. This may be in the context of challenging behaviours. It's possible the patient is exhibiting a degree of idealisation and devaluation towards different staff members, is behaving inconsistently, emotionally labile, and, therefore, unpredictably, producing an interactive dynamic where the patient finds themselves in conflict with some staff members who develop split – or different – views about the patient from colleagues, about what is causing their behaviour and how to treat them. Main was clear that these divergent views were *not caused* by the patients and could not be.

In fact, 'splitting' originally referred to a person's inability to bring together, in their thinking, the dichotomy of perceived negative and positive qualities into a cohesive whole. A defence against overwhelming or intolerable emotions, it leads to the person seeing things in absolute terms, perceiving a person or situation as either all good or all bad, idealising someone or devaluing them.

Page (2018) noted how, over time, the terminology used to describe this internal phenomenon 'has become reified and splitting has been discussed in terms that are apt to frame the process as patient-precipitated…and attribute to patients' responsibility for events that are beyond their control'.

Why is all this important? Because these myths about BPD/EUPD make it more difficult for people with the disorder to get effective treatment and help. They highlight the need for teams to have clear systems for:

- the use of care plans;
- clinical communication;
- maintaining consistency;
- continuity of care.

Regular access to clinical supervision and reflective practice should give them the collective and individual support needed in what is very challenging and emotionally intense work.

Moreover, this kind of stigmatising approach deflects from the fact that, too often, there are not effective services available to this client group and the ability of individual clinicians to adequately help the patient manage their risk is severely impeded, even though the prognosis is relatively positive when suitable treatment is available (Leib et al., 2004).

And the risk is significant. Between 60 per cent and 78 per cent of people with BPD/EUPD have experienced suicidal thoughts and more than 90 per cent have self-harmed (Biskin and Paris, 2012). Ten per cent of people with BPD will die by suicide, a rate almost 50 times that of the general population, with completed suicides more common after the age of 30 (Leib et al., 2004).

Assessing risk with BPD patients is complicated by the frequency of suicidal thoughts, and, for some, suicide attempts, as well as self-harming acts. But prospective studies indicate the predictors of suicide in patients with BPD/EUPD were reported as:

- co-occurring symptoms of dissociation;
- affective reactivity;
- self-harm;
- depression comorbidity;
- family history of suicide;
- history of childhood abuse (Kulacaoglu and Kose, 2018).

As Linehan (2019) points out, compassion for the person and finding sufficient understanding of their particular situation to validate the feelings that go with it are inherent in working with people with BPD. There are reasons for challenging behaviour, no matter how unsettling it is and unreasonable it seems, reasons for wanting the attention of clinicians and trying to get their help, even if the ways these are executed appear unhelpful and unhealthy to others. Ultimately, when trying to address the risk(s) facing them because of their traumatised state of mind, trying to understand how self-harm and even suicide can be seen as helpful and desirous by the patient is an essential step in assisting them to change their mind and come to the realisation that the alternative can be equally helpful.

Risk of dangerousness, violence and/or homicide

The key factor in violence is biological. As we shall see, and as is the case with suicide, violence and homicide are intrinsically linked to male gender. Psychology, pathology, politics and ideology all figure in violence but, overwhelmingly, in the distressing cases referred to in this section, and the statistics that demonstrate its scale and impact, we return again and again to the male gender. This is inevitably reflected in people with mental health problems, including severe mental illness, but should be seen in that context and no other significance read into it.

People with mental health problems are far more likely to be victims rather than perpetrators of violence. Again, the majority will be men. However, 'people with some types of mental disorder are more likely to be violent than others in the general population, a fact that is uncomfortable for many in the mental health sector' (Thorneycroft, 2020). Schizophrenia and bipolar disorder carry a slightly higher risk but people suffering with a combination of severe mental illness, substance misuse and anti-social personality disorder are significantly more likely to be violent than someone with severe mental illness alone (Putkonen et al., 2004).

It is an area of clinical work that can arouse high emotions amongst practitioners. Descriptive terms are often used inappropriately and in highly subjective ways, which can lead to misunderstanding, the labelling of people and unhelpful responses from staff (Repper and Perkins, 2003).

Even referring to the literature, there are varying definitions of commonly used terms. Therefore the definitions offered below should be treated with caution. It is far better to actually describe the act that has taken place rather than using generic terms e.g. 'Oliver was shouting loudly, swearing and making threats to staff. He then threw a chair across the room at Staff Nurse Murray which narrowly missed her legs', or 'Oliver shouted at Nurse Murray, saying that he would hit her if she did not leave the room but walked away without any intervention'. If generic terms such as 'anger' or 'violence' are used, the clinician should be as precise and accurate as possible when communicating with others, either orally or in documentation.

Key definitions

- **Hostility:** Exhibiting enmity or opposition, to others, objects or ideas. It can also be described as a personality trait which reflects the interpretation of others' actions as harmful and can result in anger.
- **Anger:** a normal, subjective emotional state involving physiological arousal and *associated cognitions*. The emphasis on the associated cognitions is important, as the state of physiological arousal is similar to that which occurs when people describe themselves as feeling anxious. It is the cognitive association of the state of physiological arousal and potential actions which is key and *may* lead to a violent response.
- **Aggression:** a hostile attitude and overt behaviour *intended* to inflict physical, psychological or emotional damage on another individual. There are different types of aggression:

  - **Predatory aggression:** stalking and perpetration of violence on another person.
  - **Social aggression:** unprovoked aggression that is directed at members of the same species or group for purposes of establishing dominance.
  - **Defensive aggression:** attacks delivered when an animal or person feels 'cornered' or trapped by a threatening aggressor. This is the type of aggression most commonly perpetrated against clinicians by patients and usually occurs when the person perceives they are at risk from staff or in an unsafe environment.

- **Violence:** attempts to use force to violate, inflict physical damage or harm. However, violence can then be further differentiated:

  - Reactive/hostile aggression (sometimes referred to as affective aggression) is a reaction to perceived provocation and arousal of hostility, described as a relatively primitive response to a perceived threat as a form of self defence. This type of affective aggression tends to be impulsive and relatively uncontrolled.
  - Instrumental aggression or predatory violence involves purposeful, deliberate goal directedness and planning to obtain an objective or goal where the violence or aggression is representative of more than causing physical injury and achieving an end other than threat alleviation.

- **Homicide:** Homicide means the killing of another human being, intentionally or accidentally, with or without justification. Criminal homicide occurs when a person purposely, knowingly, recklessly or negligently causes the death of another. Murder and manslaughter are both examples of criminal homicide. Manslaughter is killing with the intent for murder but where a partial defence applies, namely loss of control, diminished responsibility or killing pursuant to a suicide pact.

Mental health and the law

A criminal act, including violence or homicide perpetrated by someone with a diagnosed mental disorder, does not necessarily mean that disorder was the reason the person carried out the crime. For example, a person may have a diagnosed mental disorder for which they are being treated, such as schizophrenia, but steal a car because they want the money they would get from selling it on. Someone with a psychotic disorder might kill his partner because he is angry and loses his temper. In both cases the criminal act has no relationship to his mental disorder. However, if he killed his partner because he had a delusional belief she was the devil and just about to kill their children, and that he had to kill her to save them, there would be grounds to link his actions to his mental disorder. It is a complex legal process though one clearly defined in law. The following gives some information about key elements.

Mens rea is often described as the "mental element" in a crime. It can include what used to be known as 'malice aforethought', i.e. conscious planning or intent, as well as something culpable but less deliberate, such as recklessness or negligence. *Actus reus* in criminal law consists of all elements of a crime other than the state of mind of the defendant. In particular, *actus reus* may consist of conduct, result, a state of affairs or an omission.

A judge will decide if a person is fit to plead and stand trial but will take advice from psychiatric reports. To be assessed as being fit to plead and stand trial, the defendant must be able to do *all* of the following:

1. Understand the nature of the charges and consequent effect of the charges.
2. Decide whether to plead guilty or not guilty.
3. Exercise their right to challenge jurors.
4. Instruct counsel and solicitor so as to prepare and make a proper defence.
5. Understand and follow the course of proceedings.
6. Give evidence in their defence.

At trial, a proven link to the person's mental disorder and the crime itself must be established. A person will be considered legally insane if they were suffering from a mental disorder at the time of the offence and, *as a result*:

• did not understand what he or she was doing or
• did not know what he or she was doing was wrong or
• was unable to not commit the crime (CPS, 2022).

There is a four-stage test for diminished responsibility, of which all four elements must be proved:

1. Whether the defendant was suffering from an abnormality of mental functioning.
2. If so, whether it had arisen from a recognised medical condition.
3. If so, whether it had substantially impaired his ability either to understand the nature of his conduct or to form a rational judgment or to exercise self-control (or any combination).
4. If so, whether it provided an explanation for his conduct.

The Crown Prosecution Service states:

> To establish the common law defence of "insanity", it must be clearly proved that, at the time of committing the act, the suspect was labouring under such a "defect of reason", from a "disease of the mind", as
>
> (i) not to know the nature and quality of the act being done (a delusion, for instance where a suspect believes they are cutting a slice of bread when in fact they are cutting a throat), or,

(ii) that the suspect did not know what was being done was wrong ("wrong" meaning contrary to the law) (CPS, 2022).

'Disposals' for offenders with mental disorders, developmental disorders or neurological impairments

A range of types of sentence, or disposal, are possible for **adult** offenders who have mental disorders, developmental disorders or neurological impairments, depending on the facts of the case, the nature of the offence and other factors, including the offender's behaviour when they are unwell. The court will also consider the need to protect the public.

- **Hospital order** – the offender is detained in a hospital for treatment.
- **Guardianship order** – the offender is placed under the guardianship of local social services or an approved person.
- **Restriction order** – if making a hospital order, the Crown Court may also make a restriction order if it appears that it is necessary to do so to protect the public from serious harm. A restriction order means that aspects of an offender's sentence, such as transfer to another hospital or discharge into the community, become subject to the consent of the Secretary of State.
- **Imprisonment with hospital direction and limitation direction** – if the Crown Court decides the criteria are met for a hospital order (offenders aged 21 or over only) the court must then also consider if it would be more appropriate to pass a sentence of imprisonment with a direction that the offender is detained in hospital (a 'hospital direction') rather than in prison. A hospital direction will always be accompanied by a limitation direction, which has the same effect as a restriction order.
- **Secretary of State transfer powers** – if a sentenced prisoner becomes mentally unwell, a prison can ask the Secretary of State to give permission to transfer the prisoner to hospital (Sentencing Council, 2022).

Homicide[xiii]

The number of homicides in the UK linked to people with mental health problems is extremely small, given a population of 67 million plus. However, each one is a unique tragedy, for the victim, their family and those around them and, if the perpetrator was unwell and acting in response to symptoms of their mental disorder, it is equally tragic for them. It is for these reasons the subject has been given so much space here.

As shown below, there are serious questions about the counting of mental health related homicides, as well as how well mental health services gather data and learn lessons from homicides (McCallion and Farrimond, 2018; Markham, 2019).

To contextualise mental health homicides, we will briefly look at the wider pattern of deaths by homicide. In the early 1960s the UK homicide rate was consistently around 300 per year (6 per million population) but steadily increased to its peak of 891 (15.1 per million population) in the year ending March 2002, having grown at a faster rate than population growth over the same period.

There was then a general decrease while the population of England and Wales continued to grow (excluding the year ending March 2003, when 173 victims of Harold Shipman were recorded). It fell to a low of 8.8 per million population (434 victims) in the year ending March 2015, increased to 11.8 in the year ending March 2018 (11.8) then fell back to 9.9 per million population (612 victims) for the year ending March 2021. The 2018 figures include 31 victims of terrorist attacks and 11 victims from the Shoreham air crash.

COVID-19 restrictions coincided with changes in homicide in 2020–21. The number of victims killed in a public place fell by 27 per cent, from 350 to 255, whereas homicides in a residential setting increased by 5 per cent (from 323 to 339).

The latest international figures for comparison from The United Nations Office on Drugs and Crime (UNODC, 2019) listed 809 deaths by homicide in 2018 in the United Kingdom, a rate of 12 per million population, the same as France but more than Germany (8 per million) and Ireland (7 per million).

The figures for each UK country were:

- England and Wales – 726 (12 per million);
- Scotland – 61 (11 per million);
- Northern Ireland – 23 (12 per million).

ONS figures for England and Wales in the year ending March 2021 (612 homicides) reveal the following.

Gender

- As in previous years, over two-thirds of all victims (70 per cent) were male.
- 109 (92 per cent) of those charged with killing a female victim were male.

Age

- As in previous years, children aged under one year had the highest rate of homicide (41 per million population).
- Teenagers were the victim of 50 homicides. In 70 per cent of these teen homicides, the method of killing was a knife or sharp instrument.
- The largest percentage increase was in the number of victims under 16 years, up from 43 to 59 (a 37 per cent increase).

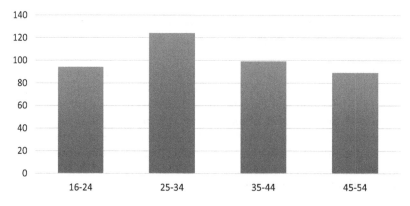

Figure 1.11 Age and number of homicide victims, 2020–2021

Crime in England and Wales: year ending March 2021 (ONS, 2021)

Ethnicity

- Over two-thirds (409 or 69 per cent) of all victims were from the White ethnic group.
- 98 victims were identified in the Black ethnic group, accounting for 16 per cent of all victims, a decrease of five homicides from the previous year.
- 48 (8 per cent) victims were in the Asian (Indian sub-continent) ethnic group.
- Ethnicity is also measured in three-year blocks for greater accuracy because of the relative low numbers. In the three years to year ending March 2021, average rates per million population were around six times higher for Black victims than White victims and almost four times higher than victims of other ethnicities.

Suspected perpetrators

- For the three-year period year ending March 2021, 995 (94 per cent) of suspects convicted of homicide were male. 40 per cent were aged 16 to 24 and 27 per cent aged 25 to 34 years. This contrasts with female suspects convicted of homicide who had an older age profile, with over half (52 per cent) being aged 35 years and over.
- Female victims were more commonly killed by a partner, ex-partner or family member. For males the suspected killer was more commonly a friend or acquaintance, stranger or other known person.
- Domestic homicides decreased by 7 to 114 (6 per cent) from the previous year, but will likely increase as police investigations continue.
- A stranger was suspected for around 18 per cent (68) of victims.
- The most common suspect in 25 of 59 (42 per cent) killings of children aged under 16 years was a parent or step-parent.

Method

- A knife or other sharp instrument was used in 235 homicides, a decrease of 13 per cent compared with the previous year, possibly due to COVID-19 restrictions.
- Over half of sharp instrument homicide victims were identified as White (60 per cent, 140 homicides). Just under a quarter (24 per cent, 57 victims) were identified as Black, a decrease of 17 compared with the previous year. Of these, 25 were aged 16 to 24 years.
- The second most common method of killing was by 'kicking or hitting', accounting for 107 homicides (18 per cent of the total). As in previous years, the majority (81 per cent) of victims killed in this way were male.

Motive

- More than half (54 per cent, 320 offences) of all homicide cases resulted from a quarrel, a revenge attack or a loss of temper, similar to previous years. This proportion was higher where the principal suspect was known to the victim (67 per cent).
- Furtherance of theft or gain accounted for 4 per cent of homicides (25 offences), and 6 per cent (38 offences) occurred during irrational acts.

Drugs and alcohol

- In the last three years 32 per cent of homicide victims were thought to be under the influence of alcohol and/or illicit drugs at the time of the homicide:

  - 18 per cent had been drinking alcohol.
  - 6 per cent had been taking an illicit drug.
  - 8 per cent were under the influence of both.

- 31 per cent of victims were known drug users.
- There were 306 homicides thought to involve drug users or dealers or in some way be drug-related.

Scotland and Northern Ireland

- In Scotland the number of victims has almost halved between 2011–2012 and 2020–2021, from 91 to 52 (17.5 to 10.6 per million population) (Scottish Government, 2022). This was the lowest number of recorded homicide cases since comparable records began in 1976.
- Northern Ireland recorded 22 homicide offences (11.6 victims per million population), one more than the previous year.

Homicide and mentally disordered offenders

Between 2009–2019, The National Confidential Inquiry into Suicide and Safety in mental Health (NCISH) was notified of 6,260 homicide convictions. Of these, 682 were patients under the care of mental health services, an average of 62 per year. The numbers peaked in 2012 at 84 and fell to 48 in 2016. However, these figures are disputed, most notably by Julian Hendy and hundredfamilies.org, which claims mental health services frequently – and sometimes deliberately — minimise the problem of violence in mental health patients, particularly homicides, and estimates the number to be an average of 120 per year.

One reason for such a huge discrepancy is that the NCISH only includes cases where the perpetrator has been in contact with secondary mental health services in the 12 months before the offence, excludes cases where the perpetrator later took his or her own life as well and, therefore, was not charged and/or convicted. Because they count the number of perpetrators convicted of homicide rather than victims, the number of people killed will be higher than the recorded homicides, as there are occasional cases of multiple homicide.

McCallion and Farrimond (2018) were commissioned by NHS England to undertake a review of the Independent Investigations for Mental Health Homicides (IIMHH) in England from 2013 to 2017.

They reviewed 57 reports. Of these, 35 were published and 22 unpublished. They concluded the IIMHH reports were variable in quality and did not in all cases meet expected standards. They were unable to establish if the recommendations of the IIMHH reports had been implemented, and if changes to policy and the embedding of learning was occurring in the NHS at local level or even if the outcomes of the IIMHH reports informed NHS England commissioning.

Again, they were unable to discern whether or not the perpetrator outline in mental health related homicides, which they had discovered through their review, had previously been identified and disseminated. But, as a result of their own review, McCallion and Farrimond (2018) noted the emerging perpetrator outline demonstrated that the majority were:

- male (80 per cent);
- in the community (95 per cent);
- known to their victims (83 per cent);
- not held under the MHA (93 per cent);
- had a median age of 36 years;
- had used legal or illegal substances (85 per cent);
- had a forensic history (58 per cent) or a history of violence (16 per cent);
- may have more than one diagnosis including: substance misuse; paranoid schizophrenia, anxiety and depression and personality disorder (64 per cent).

Other factors are known about people with mental health problems who were perpetrators of homicide. The research programme based at the University of Manchester stated in an earlier report on 662 patient homicides between 2004–2014 (NCISH, 2016):

- 276 (49 per cent) perpetrators were either non-adherent with drug treatment in the month before the homicide or had missed their last contact with services, meaning that they were not receiving their planned treatment.
- 74 per cent experienced alcohol misuse, 78 per cent experienced drug misuse and 25 per cent experienced severe mental health problems (including schizophrenia and affective disorders) and co-morbid alcohol/drug abuse.
- Homicides committed by someone with a history of schizophrenia numbered 6 per cent, while 4 per cent were carried out by someone with a history of personality disorder, without co-morbid alcohol/drug abuse.
- Most perpetrators were:

  - male (86 per cent);
  - not currently married (79 per cent);
  - unemployed (83 per cent) and
  - had a history of violence (52 per cent);
  - had previous convictions (78 per cent).

The prevalence of schizophrenia in the population is 1 per cent or less. As noted above, though the numbers are extremely small, the at least six-fold prevalence of all homicides by people with schizophrenia is an important finding that correlates with other studies that have highlighted the relationship between schizophrenia and violence, albeit one which is not as strong as that between substance misuse, alcohol or personality disorder with violence. It emphasises the need to actively treat psychotic symptoms when those are linked to the risk of violence (Maden, 2007). It's also important to emphasise that mental ill health increases the risk of violence and homicide but is not the cause.

Key risk factors in patient homicide include:

1. An identified risk of dangerousness.
2. A history of violence.
3. Experiencing psychotic symptoms e.g. delusional beliefs, command hallucinations.
4. Misusing drugs and alcohol.
5. Non attendance of appointments.
6. Non compliance with treatment.
7. The presence of other psychotic symptoms.

Nonetheless, even when those factors were present in the history of patients who went on to commit homicide, at final service contact:

- 88 per cent of people were assessed as no immediate or 'low risk';
- 1 per cent were assessed as being 'high risk' (Appleby et al., 2006).

Violent crime in the UK

Violent crime in England and Wales rose steadily from the year ending March 2010 (367,847 recorded crimes of violence with injury) to 549,645 in 2018. After two years of decline it reached a new high of 566,603 in the year to March 2021. These crimes ranged from attempted murder, which trebled between 2011–12 and 2016–17 when it peaked at 1,343 before settling at just over 1,000 per year, and actual bodily harm (ONS, 2022).

Table 1.6 Risk factors in aggression and/or violence

Historical	Cognitive	Mental health diagnosis	Verbal
Genetic (family heredity) factors	Ruminating on angry feelings and events	Misuse of drugs and/or alcohol	Denying or minimising dangerous acts
Being the victim of physical abuse and/or sexual abuse	Preoccupation with violent fantasy	Antisocial personality disorder	Expressing intent/ threats to harm others
Exposure to violence in the home and/or community	Suspicious and/or perceiving threat from others	Autism/Asperger's syndrome plus complex needs	Describing angry and/ or uncontrollable feelings
Early age at first violence	**Emotions**	Traumatic brain injury	Increased volume of speech
Previous aggression/violence	Anxiety/fear	Psychosis	**Behavioural**
Previous use of weapons	Anger	Dementia	Increased physical arousal
Previous dangerous, impulsive acts	Hostility	**Specific symptoms**	Exaggerated reactions
Exposure to violence in media	Frustration	Violent command hallucinations	Invasion of body space
Known personal trigger factors	Suspicion	Paranoid delusions about others	Being sexually inappropriate
Previous admissions to secure settings	Lack of guilt/remorse about offending behaviour	Morbid jealousy	Facial tension
Previously in prison	Dependency on recognition by others	Passivity	Associating with delinquent peers
Other			
Male gender, especially under 35 years of age	Unstable living arrangements	Recent discontinuation of, or non compliance with, medication	Relationship instability
Exposure to violence in media	Employment/financial problems	Non attendance of appointments	Presence of firearms in home
Combination of stressful family socioeconomic factors (poverty, severe deprivation, parental breakup, poor parenting, unemployment, loss of support from extended family)			

Analysis from 2016–17 highlights male involvement in violent crime and the proportionate increase associated with the severity of brutality. Males account for:

- 85 per cent of assailants of common assault;
- 88 per cent of actual bodily harm;
- 91 per cent of grievous bodily harm (the latter resulting in serious injuries to the victim, such as broken bones or permanent disfigurement);
- 98 per cent of sexual offending (Das, 2019).

Scotland saw its violent crime halve to 6,272 between 2008–2009 and 2014–2015, after which it rose to 9,316 in 2019–2020, falling back slightly to 8,972 in 2020–2021 (Scottish Government 2022).

In Northern Ireland there were 29,328 recorded crimes of violence against the person in 2010–2011. By 2019–2020 this had risen to 41,305 before dropping to 39,204 the following year.

The relationship between mental illness and violence

Substance misuse has a far greater effect on crime and homicide than mental health. It has been estimated that 'heroin and crack cocaine, along with the recent explosion in New Psychoactive Substances, drive as much as 50 per cent of all acquisitive crime, and 70 per cent of shop thefts' while there were 73,661 drug related robberies. Police recorded shop theft cases of more than 385,000 offences in 2017 but the true figure, based on Home Office assumptions, is closer to 38 million offences (Centre for Social Justice, 2018).

As demonstrated above, the trend across the UK has been for an increase in violent crime over the last decade or so. There is no similar statistical database related to violence from people with a mental disorder. However, Senior et al. (2020) calculated that 53 per cent of all violent incidents in England and Wales in 2015–2016 were perpetrated by people with severe mental illness – at a total annual cost to society of £2.5 billion.

There is older evidence that the prevalence of violence of people diagnosed with schizophrenia is higher (8 per cent) than that in the general population (2 per cent), but with a far higher relationship between alcohol abuse and violence (24 per cent), and those people drug dependent engaging in violent behaviour (34 per cent) (Swanson et al., 1997). Women who suffer from psychiatric illness have higher rates of violence than women in the general population (Stueve and Link, 1998).

The United States Justice Department reported that people with a history of mental illness but not abusing drugs or alcohol were responsible for 4.3 per cent of homicides. That figure rose to 25 per cent where the homicide was that of a parent (Allnutt et al., 2010).

The significance of the presence of psychotic symptoms is fully discussed by Allnutt et al. (2010), who note that the risk of violence increases in cases where the person's symptoms are not being treated, particularly if this is due to the patient refusing treatment. Violent offences are often linked to delusional beliefs.

According to Hodgins (2008), among violent offenders with schizophrenia there are three distinct types who are defined by the age of onset of antisocial and violent behaviour:

- Type 1: 'Early starters' display pattern of antisocial behaviour that emerges in childhood or early adolescence, well before the onset of any illness. Their violence tends to remain stable across their lifespan.
- **Type 2:** Constitutes the largest group of violent offenders with schizophrenia. They show no antisocial behaviour prior to the onset of the illness then repeatedly engage in aggressive behaviour towards others.
- **Type 3:** A small number display a chronic course of schizophrenia with no aggressive behaviour for 1–2 decades after illness onset then engage in serious violence, often killing those who care for them.

However, there is, generally, no close association between aggressive behaviour and positive symptoms of psychosis. Aggressive behaviour tends to reflect a lack of interpersonal skills and poor psychosocial functioning. Hodgins (2008) noted psychosocial functioning was associated with two static predictors: the person's level of education and past diagnoses of substance misuse disorders and three current predictors, these being the presence of depression, non-compliance with antipsychotic medication and experiences of physical victimisation.

Inpatient settings, by their very nature, accommodate disturbed/distressed and often challenging patients, many of whom don't want to be there and where problems as a consequence of psychotic phenomena are most acutely experienced. Several UK studies have found numbers of inpatients who have perpetrated violence to be as high as 28–32 per cent. Daffern et al. (2007) noted:

> Staff's refusal of requests or demands of activity are often perceived by patients as annoying, unfair, disrespectful, unjust, frustrating or irritating. Aggression towards staff and patients seems to be commonly preceded by frustration and often appeared to have a tension reducing quality.

Key clinical tip

Re-assessment of individual patients in an inpatient unit is required not just when observable change occurs in that person's behaviour or their circumstances but when factors in the ward environment occur which could destabilise them, no matter how previously stable they have been.

The pathway to violence

As with suicide, the same question remains after studying statistics and all the other information about violence and dangerous behaviour directed at others. Why do some people who have experienced a lot of the traumas and potential risk factors set out in this section, especially those set out in Table 1.6, never hurt anyone else? What differentiates those people – the majority – who can turn those setbacks into something that motivates them positively from those who turn to violence? Crucially, as noted by Sinai et al. (2017), there is a similarity to those people who attempt to end their life with suicidal intent:

1. Traumatising triggering events or enabling conditions in the person's environment.
2. A lack of perceived alternatives to engaging in violence to redress grievance(s) due to their psychological disposition.
3. The capability to embark on violent action.
4. The absence of internal and external protective factors to preempt or prevent such violence.

The authors created a model explaining the pathway to violence synthesized from 'existing concepts and models found in academic, government, and law enforcement literature'. Their interest was in looking at 'progressively escalating risk-based mindsets and behaviours by susceptible individuals that culminate in a violent active-shooter type attack', what are commonly described as 'mass shootings' but can be applied to 'other types of violent actors' (Sinai et al., 2017).

Models such as this attempt to detail a pathway, or stages, an individual may travel before actually responding to perceived grievances and injustices, using violence in ways which are reactive/hostile, often impulsively and relatively uncontrolled or predatory. It is purposeful, goal directed and planned to obtain an objective or goal where the violence or aggression is representative of more than causing physical injury and achieving an end other than threat alleviation.

They acknowledged it was for use as a training and reference resource. Pathway to violence models are intended to support analysts and clinicians by outlining risk based factors that *might* lead to violence but 'should not be considered as diagnostically valid for clinical purposes' (Sinai et al., 2017).

The question about why everyone doesn't complete this pathway and act violently seems, again, to have a similarity to suicide. Most individuals have protective factors. Angry thoughts, mindsets and even behaviours don't usually progress to actual violence against other people. Even well developed fantasies about being violent – sometimes in quite explicit, carefully thought through ways – don't always translate into action. This can be for all kinds of reasons, e.g. the fear of consequences, a moral code about what is right and wrong, a sense of how others would perceive us if we were violent, an empathic sense of the impact of the imagined act upon the victim. It might be that others intervene and prevent the violence, or something happens that breaks the cognitive and emotional pattern that was leading the individual on their pathway to violence, enabling them to change the outcome for themselves.

The same kind of protective factors that protect us from suicidal thoughts will be evident in avoiding overt violence, including a strong social support network, particularly from caring family members, positive social connections and involvement with others, a willingness to seek help and openness to it and resilient personality traits, particularly those developed in early years.

It is when these fail and/or an individual's maladaptive or negative coping mechanisms prevail, that a threshold is crossed, and actual violence is more likely to result from an individual's grievances, fantasies and planning.

The elements that lead to the diminishing of these protective factors and crossing of this threshold are complex and varied. For many, it may be through acquiring the capability for violence, in much the same way as Selby and Joiner (2009) postulate that people acquire the capability to end their life. This can be through direct exposure to physical violence. There are theories that exposure to violence on TV or through video games can be the gateway. Some others might acquire it through reading and study of the subject.

The case of John LaDue, a 17 year old schoolboy from a small town in Minnesota is revealing. He was arrested after being found to have a storage locker equipped with bomb making equipment, ammunition and weapons. In his home he had almost 180 pages of notes, his plans laid out, and a semi automatic rifle, two handguns and three ready made explosive devices. In summary:

> He would use a .22-caliber rifle to "dispose of" his mother, father and sister. He would set a brushfire outside of town to occupy first responders. Then he would head to Waseca Junior/Senior High School, plant a couple of pressure cooker bombs, and wait for students to stream out between classes. He would remotely detonate the bombs before walking through the school, guns blasting. He would shoot locks off classroom doors and toss small bombs into rooms filled with his frightened peers. When police arrived, he would confront them, too. He assumed he would die from their fire.
>
> (Louwagie, 2017)

Asked by the police officer interrogating him, "Why would you dispose of your family? What have they done?" LaDue replied, "They did nothing wrong. I just wanted as many victims as possible."

At the time, everyone was baffled. John had no history of violence. No history of mental health problems. No overt or obvious trauma. No apparent interest in violence. His friends were 'ordinary' and 'normal'. He said, "I have good parents. I live in a good town." His parents were loving, kind, caring. The evening of his arrest they were frantically trying to find him because he was never out late on a school night.

Before going to trial, John went through interviews with psychologists using various assessment tools for violence, psychopathy and mental illness. None raised a red flag. All three psychologists who assessed him concluded he had autistic spectrum disorder and had been stuck in 'grievance-oriented thinking', focusing on retribution towards people and institutions he believed had been dismissive of him, treated him unfairly and failed to appreciate his greatness, viewing some of his peers as so stupid and immature they had no right to live.

It also emerged that John had immersed himself in the history of mass killings, in schools and elsewhere, critiquing the killers, their methods and outcomes in fine detail, including the most effective into his plans, discarding the ones that had the least impact, i.e. number of deaths.

Yet, through this alone, John LaDue struggled to cross the threshold. He had planned the massacre for April 2014 but was arrested on April 29th. Questioned about this he described several reasons he hadn't acted. It emerged everything was meticulously planned except the launching of the attack. He had other reasons not to proceed, such as needing to steal a shotgun, get more ammunition. He'd even set off a small explosion in the playground then put a letter in someone's mailbox, asking them to pass it on to the police. They never did. But John said afterwards he wanted 'a check from a psychiatrist', to discover 'what's wrong with me actually'.

There was a further twist. John LaDue could only be charged with possession of explosives as he hadn't acted upon his ideas and couldn't be charged for things he had thought about but not enacted. He was released after two years in juvenile facilities, initially on probation and with mandatory sessions with a psychiatrist. However, after deciding to plead guilty to the felony charge of possession of explosives, he was completely free and continued to reintegrate himself into his local community. By this point he had been diagnosed with narcissistic personality disorder, unspecified personality disorder and having had a major depressive episode, a diagnosis that made more sense to him.

Inevitably the subject of huge curiosity, he opened up to two journalists working on different articles. In an interview published online, he talked of increasing irritability with other children who were 'messing around' during his seventh and eighth grade years. "I felt like I should have been doing better than I was," he said.

> There wasn't a distinct pushing moment. It was just a gradual build... I wasn't enjoying things. I looked around and people were enjoying stuff, and I was just living day to day, just existing. So it was more fuelled by my disappointment and frustration that led me to want to be violent, it's because I wanted to feel satisfaction through dominance, basically.
>
> (wbur, 2018)

Pam Louwagie (2017) described how John was able to explain, two years on, setting 'impossible standards for himself', growing frustrated and depressed when failing to meet them: 'it bothered him that his German teacher knew more about the language than he did. If Mozart composed music at age 5, why couldn't he master a guitar riff?' Expanding on his comments in the online interview John described wanting respect and imagining fear and surprise on the faces of his victims as he pointed his gun at them. "I just wanted to hold their lives in my hand," he explained.

Had more of the risk factors identified in Table 1.6 been present in John's case, might he have acted earlier? Might he be another name in the infamous list of school shooters? Looking at the KGH Pathway to Violence model (Table 1.7) is a useful way of assessing what drove him on to acquire the weapons and plan his attack but might have stopped him crossing the threshold, whether temporarily or not.

Table 1.7 A modified version of The KGH Pathway to Violence Model (2017)

1	Cognitive opening	Conscious and unconscious mental and psychological predispositions which foster: • adaptive responses i.e. coping responses and strategies to reduce stress and are protective, or • maladaptive responses to traumatic events, crises and/or stressors which are unhealthy, neurotic and, in extreme cases, can have an intensity that increases the likelihood of the individual using violence to address perceived grievances.
2	Triggering events	Often traumatic, the event or events angers and aggravates the perpetrator. Rather than one event it is more likely to be a series or 'cumulative process', a final triggering event being the catalyst. These might include: • failures at school/work and/or personal relationships; • portrayals of violence in social media; • propagation of extremist ideologies and role models; • peer encouragement; • psychotic symptoms including delusional beliefs and/or auditory hallucinations.

Table 1.7 (Continued)

3	Grievance	The person is left with a sense of grievance from the triggering events.
4	Ideation/Fantasy	The act of forming ideas. These may include thinking of how to put ideas into action, engaging in a violent act and harming someone/others. Importantly, the authors include the possibility of suicidal as well as homicidal ideation. A number of perpetrators of homicide will describe having thought about their own death before deciding to kill someone else, possibly experiencing suicidal thoughts after the crime. This stage is also likely to include collecting examples of other perceived injustices, focusing on 'perceived grievances, destructive envy, and a nurturing of feelings of persecution'.
5	Planning	The person begins to develop a plan to engage in a violent act to harm someone/others. It's important to note at this point that the nature of the violence, i.e. reactionary or predatory, will depend on other personality traits and cognitive, emotional and situational factors. This is likely to be accompanied by social withdrawal, target selection, thinking about the time and place and possible threats being made.
6	Preparation	The person begins making specific preparations to carry out their plan to harm someone/others. This might include procuring weapons or the means, and possibly practicing.
7	Implementation	The person acts on their plan and preparations by perpetrating violence upon someone/others.

While Sinai et al. (2017) were primarily concerned with school shooters, we can still consider the application of this model to a patient in a forensic unit who perceives himself treated unjustly by being incarcerated for a lengthy period under the Mental Health Act when his criminal offence would have warranted a very short custodial sentence at most. Adding to this, not considering himself unwell, he believes he's been unfairly detained. With a long history of trauma, neglect, difficulties at school and poor interpersonal relationships, he now feels particularly disrespected by a fellow patient. He ruminates on his situation and starts to think about how he might seek retribution. Wanting to inflict a high degree of violence but limited in his choice of weapons he decides upon boiling water mixed with sugar. He then waits for an opportune moment when he can put the water and sugar in a cup, go to the other patient's room at a time the door is open and there will be minimal risk of intervention from the staff and throw it in his face.

Equally, it can be used to understand the reactionary violence from a person with a longstanding substance misuse problem, attending the Emergency Department after self-harming, who feels frustrated and angry at what they perceive to be the uncaring attitude of staff who are busy with other patients. With a deep sense of grievance, mixed with shame and anxiety related to early trauma and neglect, he ruminates on his current situation but finds it hard to disentangle it from historic grievances and past traumas. Looking around, he sees a chair, thinks that would make a suitable weapon and throws it at the screen in front of the triage nurse who has asked him to wait.

As with those who attempt or complete the act of suicide, the person preparing an act of violence may let clues about their intention leak out, whether consciously or unconsciously, with attempts to seek help through often very indirect or abstract ways. It will depend on a variety of factors, such as the individual's psychopathology, family and social support, understanding of the potential impact on others and history of help-seeking behaviour and protective factors. Conversely, the more adverse, maladaptive stress responses and negative coping mechanisms, the less likely the person will be to seek help or for potential clues to their intention to leak out.

It is inevitable that there will be far less time for any intervention if the person adopts a reactive response.

Shame and violence

Shame has long been known to be a precursor to violence. However, it is often hard to address within an assessment. Most people want to avoid talking about or acknowledging anything that could give rise to even further feelings of shame. Submissive behaviour, avoidance and concealment are prime mechanisms for managing one's feelings of shame. Moreover, the nature of shame – self-focused, defence-orientated – doesn't lend itself to pro-social behaviours. It can broadly be defined as having three separate sources:

1. a violation of an accepted standard or role;
2. a failure to meet expectations;
3. a defect of the self that cannot easily be repaired (Poulson, 2001).

It is important, therefore, to develop an understanding of what shame is, how it affects us and how it might result in violence. Clinicians can then think about what to look for and how to broach the subject in a way that allows the person to discuss it.

As anyone reading this will know from their own experience, people try to hide from anything shaming – and hide it from others – to get away from whatever caused the feeling. These actions can restore a feeling of being in control in response to a situation where control seems to have been lost. In this way, shame has been advanced as a useful response to difficulty. It can help us remedy problems, progress and improve, e.g. working harder academically after the shame of failing an exam (Deonna et al., 2011).

Thomason (2015) has described shame as arising out of 'a tension between our identity and self conception': we feel ashamed of things that are part of our identities, but not part of how we see ourselves. Shame, she argues, is a result of some aspect of our identity becoming all encompassing. It comes to define us, dominating everything we experience. Thus, the teenager who fails an exam feels that aspect of their identity becomes prominent, is what everyone knows about them and defines them as a whole. It contrasts with our self conception, or the self image of how we 'represent to ourselves the person we take ourselves to be'. In this case, not someone who fails exams.

However, the inability to reject that part of the self by which the person feels shame can have the doubly disabling effect of leaving them feeling powerless.

It is not just because we fail to live up to an idealised version of ourselves. It occurs when, contrary to what we thought of our moral code or moral character, we prove ourselves capable of actions we thought we would never do, that we know or believe to be 'wrong'.

Henrikson (2020) notes how shame can be defined to issues like race and gender, totally beyond the individual's control, giving rise to the feeling that they are wholly defined by their skin colour or sex and how others perceive them because of that.

In philosophical literature there have been doubts cast on the idea that anyone would respond to a feeling of shame by doing something perhaps even more shameful, i.e. perpetrating an act of violence against another person. Henrikson (2020) notes this often ignores how irrational shame can be, and how some people are 'shame-prone', often with a maladaptive self image, and talks about the interruption of an intentional action with a desired, positive outcome that engenders shame, which is more than an experience of failure to achieve the desired good. It may comprise an experience of failure or lack of ability to act in ways that can lead to the desired result. It may be an experience of the desire or intention itself as failed, or as considered by others as objectionable. This results in reduced self esteem and self worth which 'may accumulate over time until a point of overload is reached'. It is this overload that seems most associated with violence (Poulson, 2001). As it accumulates, every shame experience focuses the person on incapacity, deficit, failure, what they might perceive as their worst possible self.

James Gilligan, a prison psychotherapist who worked with, and studied, violent men, studying the interactions that occurred around violent incidents, was one of the first to highlight the link between shame and violence. Gilligan (1997) concluded violence was most often 'provoked by the experience of feeling shamed and humiliated, disrespected and ridiculed, and ... represented the attempt to prevent or undo this "loss of face" – no matter how severe the punishment', but noted the experience of feelings of shame on their own was not sufficient to explain violent behaviour. He described three preconditions:

1. 'Probably the most closely guarded secret held by violent men', Gilligan wrote, 'is that they feel ashamed', noting nothing is more shameful than to feel ashamed.
2. Violent men perceive themselves as having no nonviolent means of warding off or diminishing their feelings of shame or low self esteem.
3. The person also 'lacks the emotional capacities or feelings which normally inhibit the violent impulses that stimulated by shame' (Gilligan 1997).

Reacting to shame with violence can allow the person to feel as if they are once more defined by their self conception, to regain the feeling that they are more than their failure, their race or gender or fears. Anger, aggression and violence can achieve the same outcome of putting the person back in control, covering up the feelings of shame and situation that created it. The violence restores a sense of agency and denies the sense of powerlessness arising from an inability to reject that part of our identity which experienced the shame in the first place. It 'instigates the one who performs it as something else and more than what he is in his shame' and one painful act that will numb the experience of another, different pain, despite the risk of creating a situation where the person is diminished in the eyes of others and creating even more shame (Henrikson, 2020).

Does shame, in part, explain the actions of John LaDue, the young man who set 'impossible standards for himself' and grew frustrated and depressed when failing to meet them? He felt that 'I should have been doing better than I was', and said, "I wasn't enjoying things. I looked around and people were enjoying stuff, and I was just...existing." Wanting to be violent 'was more fuelled by my disappointment and frustration'. Violence, he thought, would give him a feeling of 'satisfaction through dominance', of having the lives of others in his hand (wbur, 2018).

Similar accounts can be found in the histories of people such as Thomas Watt Hamilton, who shot and killed sixteen primary children and their teacher in a school in Dunblane, and Kipland Kinkel, a fifteen-year-old who shot and killed his father, a highly respected but retired teacher at the high school Kip attended, and after telling his mother he loved her, killed her too. The next day he drove to Thurston High School, went to the school cafeteria and opened fire with the rifle he had hidden under a long coat, killing two and wounding 25. He was overpowered after running out of ammunition. After his trial he was sentenced to 112 years in prison. Both killers provided ample evidence of shame experiences throughout their lives in accounts written prior to their violent acts (Poulson, 2001).

In a different context but still examining shame, Retzinger (1991), identified what she termed 'code words' and phrases that gave clues to feelings of shame experienced by the speaker and its context. They can be broken down into the following groups:

1. Direct indication – 'I feel humiliated', 'I'm embarrassed' etc.
2. Abandonment, separation, statements about feeling isolated or indications of not belonging.
3. Ridicule – words or phrases about feeling hurt, put down, threatened by another person etc.
4. Inadequate – statements about not measuring up to one's own or others' standards.
5. Discomfort – references to unease in social settings.
6. Confused/indifferent – statements that indicate a muddled thought process.

As we shall see, risk assessment utilises the decoding of the language of the potentially violent person and explores their experience in ways that allow them to give as clear an account as possible of their feelings and how they are trying to manage them. Risk management is part of a process that attempts to help the person find adaptive, healthy ways to respond to these powerful feelings in a safe, nonviolent way.

Threat control override

Threat control override (TCO) has long been regarded as 'the propensity to overestimate the likelihood that an outside agent will (1) inflict harm (threat) or (2) control one's behaviours (control-override)' (Fanning et al., 2011). It has been associated with aggression in both people with a psychiatric disorder and those in the general population. The authors looked at this phenomena and also explored whether or not those people in the general population who were more prone to developing a psychotic disorder – given they are much larger in numbers than people with an actual, diagnosed psychotic disorder – were also likely to experience the same phenomena.

After a detailed study of 60 men and 60 women with no history of psychotic disorders, they concluded 'psychosis proneness ... is associated with increased aggressive behaviour. Furthermore, this relationship is at least partially mediated through the threat experiences, such that psychosis proneness is associated with a greater tendency to feel threatened, which in turn is associated with a greater tendency to act out aggressively'. This perceived – or real – threat is seen as a provocation that elicits aggressive behaviour.

However, while they concurred with earlier research that the experience of feeling threatened was heightened in both people who were psychotic and prone to becoming psychotic, the relationship to 'control-override' was more questionable and 'it's possible the relationship between control-override and aggression depends on the presence of other factors, such as impairments in executive functioning or cognitive disorganisation' (Fanning et al., 2011). There does seem to be a link between symptoms of threat to the severity of the violence – but not control-override – and those with paranoid delusions and related psychotic symptoms are more likely to be perpetrators of more severe violence (Stompe et al., 2004).

It's important to remind ourselves that most individuals with these symptoms are not going to be violent and pose no risk to others, while the relative risk lies in more common factors, such as male gender and substance abuse. Nonetheless, the potential for violence and threat perception needs to be assessed, including the identification of any aggressive or violent behaviours present before the onset of any mental disorder. These then need to be addressed, alongside targeted, proactive interventions to treat the person's psychosis. The risk management plan will aim to reduce the potential for aggressive or violent behaviours, especially in response to perceived threat.

Specific to managing violence, four factors need to be considered (see also Part 5, Developing a risk management plan):

- **Risk history** – this needs to be understood, particularly in relation to its impact on dynamic risk factors, but is about static risk factors that cannot be affected.
- **Current context** – how can you change the situation and/or circumstances around the person and dynamic risk factors affecting them?
- **Physiological state of arousal** – how can you reduce this and calm the person?
- **The psychological interpretation of the state of the arousal** – what can you do to change the person's thinking and perception of the situation?

Risk assessment in prisons and forensic services

Prisons

The environment

People with a mental illness in the Criminal Justice System (CJS) have been described by Public Health England as an 'underserved' population. Services are not appropriate or accessible to them due to personal and structural barriers such as 'stigma, low levels of help-seeking behaviour or complex commissioning arrangements leading to fragmented pathways, as well as challenging personal and social circumstances' – as noted by a joint thematic inspection of the criminal justice journey for individuals with mental health needs and disorders (HMIP, 2021).

Despite improvements in prison healthcare since 2005, when the NHS took over responsibility for healthcare in prisons, the Commons Select Committee (HoC, 2021) noted much greater progress is required to overcome a multitude of longstanding problems. The Committee highlighted the need for urgent action to prevent mentally ill people being sent to or kept in prison due to a shortage of mental health services in the community (HoC , 2021). Put another way, prison is a ripe incubator for the depressive symptoms, despair, anxiety and dysfunction that fuel self-harm, suicide and violence.

The problems for those suffering severe mental health problems in prison are further compounded not just by the unsuitability of the environment but also the shortage of beds in NHS secure psychiatric hospitals. A 2022 Freedom of Information Act request revealed that more than half the 5,403 prisoners in England 'assessed by prison-based psychiatrists to require hospitalisation were not transferred between 2016 and 2021 – an 81 per cent increase on the number of prisoners denied a transfer in the previous five years' (Wall, 2022). The already complex and challenging task of assessing and managing risk is, then, even more difficult in this context. The patient group is detained, most often against its will. Different legislative frameworks from psychiatric and community settings are used, with specific sections of the Mental Health Act used to detain patients in forensic units. The Act doesn't apply in prisons at all, although the Conservative Government has stated it 'planned to change the Mental Health Act to ensure people in the criminal justice system could get the right care', and there is currently a reliance on The Mental Capacity Act (Wall, 2022).

As noted, the risk management plan for patients suffering serious mental health problems but unwilling to accept treatment cannot solely rest on transferring the person to a forensic unit outside of prison. Clinicians can't rely on imposing treatment against the patient's will. But even those patients collaborating with staff and who might benefit from transfer to hospital can find themselves 'stuck' inside prison or facing lengthy delays before transfer even when accepted. Box 5 highlights different factors about prison that have a detrimental effect on mental health.

Box 5:   Factors about prison that impact on the prisoner's mental health

- The loss of support networks, particularly family and carers.
- A perceived loss of control of every aspect of their life. It is clear some things are lost, e.g. one's physical freedom, being locked up, having to wait for someone to unlock doors in order to go anywhere inside the prison, having to obey officers' instructions at all times.
- Being unable to do things most people would take for granted, such as choosing their food, how to spend their leisure time, what to wear.
- Having limited access to activities, particularly more healthy coping mechanisms when stressed, such as going for a walk or particular types of exercise, quiet time.
- Huge limitations on privacy, with very little choice about mixing with other prisoners, particularly their cell mate(s).
- The environment itself, particularly in the older Victorian prisons, with overcrowded cells, poor facilities, lots of noise and lack of space for suitable healthcare facilities.
- The 'regime' in prison, whereby the discipline staff, or prison officers, maintain a schedule to try and ensure every prisoner has access to meals, exercise, a shower, employment, education and association or social time together which means everything is done in a regimented way.
- The regime and the discipline staff's objectives often being in direct contrast with the prisoner's healthcare needs, e.g. being locked in a cell and not accessible to a healthcare practitioner when the practitioner is available, there being no officers available to escort a prisoner for an outpatient appointment in an outside hospital or clinic.
- Chronic staffing shortages, of both officers and healthcare staff, meaning the regime cannot be fully provided and prisoners' basic needs are not consistently met.
- The way in which services are commissioned can sometimes result in healthcare being fragmented and lacking cohesion, e.g. different service providers for primary care, mental health, substance misuse and separate GP services etc. This can lead to healthcare providers struggling to maintain consistency and continuity in care for individual patients.

> • Communications between the various groups in the prison, e.g. discipline staff, different healthcare providers, can be poor, exacerbated by the prison and health-care services using different electronic record keeping systems.
> • Systems that are inadequate for the task, e.g. reception screening templates[xiv] that nurses cannot realistically complete in the allotted time they have, or Mental Health Inreach Teams[xv] whose individual members have larger caseloads than they should because the teams are not funded to meet the demand from within the prison.

However, the 'problem' of undertaking an adequate reception screening in the time available is not the real issue. It is that not enough nurses are allocated to the task. Whatever the reason for that, it can result in prisoners with multiple health problems not having those problems identified and addressed. Risk indicators can be easily missed, and the prisoner can be 'lost' to the system post reception. As is the case in many community settings, the person can be subjected to multiple assessments and, as already noted, then have several different practitioners involved in their treatment and care who may not be in regular contact with one another and who lack established forums in which to discuss the person's care.

There is very limited space for confidential access to patients inside prison and limitations on the amount of time prisoners are available to clinicians, making it even more difficult to establish a rapport and then develop a therapeutic relationship. Probing into what are likely to be very intimate and sensitive issues is inevitably complicated by the same issues. Talking to someone through a small hatch in their cell door while stood on an echoey landing inevitably makes it extremely difficult to achieve the necessary intimacy required for a full risk assessment.

The prisoner

Arriving into this environment are an already vulnerable and at risk group. It has been estimated on different occasions that up to 90 per cent of prisoners meet the diagnostic criteria for at least one mental disorder, while 70 per cent had two or more disorders and 11.7 per cent met the criteria for five disorders (see, for example Singleton et al., 1998 and Bebbington et al., 2017). Looking at the figures in more detail:

- 9.2 per cent of male prisoners and 5 per cent of females have previously been admitted to a psychiatric hospital;
- 22 per cent of men and almost 29 per cent of women said they had been in contact with mental health services in the year before custody;
- most prisoners experience common conditions, e.g. depression or anxiety;
- 12–16 per cent of men in prison have reported symptoms indicative of psychosis (compared with the rate among the general public of about 4 per cent, with 1 per cent diagnosed with schizophrenia);
- 25 per cent have been diagnosed with attention deficit hyperactivity disorder;
- 7 per cent had a learning disability and 2–4 per cent diagnosed as having autistic spectrum disorder;
- 8 per cent had PTSD;
- 33 per cent and 57 per cent respectively were alcohol and drug dependent (Singleton et al., 1998; Bebbington et al., 2017 and Durcan, 2021).

Young people in custody have an even greater prevalence of poor mental health:

- 95 per cent of 16–20-year-olds are estimated to have at least one mental health problem;
- 80 per cent have more than one disorder (Lader et al., 2000);
- few have any qualifications;
- 80% have experienced temporary exclusion from school, with 58% having been permanently expelled (Williams, 2015);
- prior to their imprisonment, many young people had traumatic experiences, such as:
  - bereavement;
  - sexual abuse or
  - violence in the home.
- Young males are 18 times more likely to commit suicide in custody than in the community (Prison Reform Trust, 2014).

In surveys conducted for prison inspection reports, completed by 8,831 prisoners across 50 prisons, published between 1 April 2019 and 30 June 2020, the following was found (HMIP, 2021):

- 36 per cent of prisoners in men's prisons and 54 per cent in women's prisons reported feeling depressed on arrival;
- 12 per cent of prisoners in men's prisons and 26 per cent in women's prisons reported feeling suicidal on arrival;
- 24 per cent of prisoners in men's prisons and 40 per cent in women's prisons reported having other mental health problems on arrival;
- 48 per cent of prisoners in men's prisons and 70 per cent in women's prisons reported having mental health problems.

Risk factors specific to prison

When looking at the risk of suicide specific to prison, the process of assessment is essentially the same. However, different risk factors have to be factored in:

- Early days in custody is the period of greatest risk for suicide. This is often defined as the first 30 days but the risk is highest in the first week, when half of early days in custody deaths occur. This is the same for newly admitted prisoners *and those transferred from other prisons.*
- Friday night and at weekends and any other times when there is may be no access to records.
- If the person has received a long sentence or been charged/convicted of certain offences, i.e. murder/manslaughter or sexual offences.
- In 2021, prisoners aged 50–59 had the highest rate of self-inflicted deaths, at a rate of 1.32 per 1,000 prisoners.
- White men are twice as likely to end their life as BAME men.
- UK nationals are more likely to end their life than foreign nationals.

Risk has to be understood as being not just about individuals or even that vulnerable people are in prison. The type of prison and the status of prisoners can also increase risk.

For example, remand prisoners, category 'A' prisoners and those in 'local' jails or young offenders institutions are more at risk of self-harm. Prisoners who were on remand (1.66 per 1,000 prisoners) had a higher rate of self-inflicted deaths than those serving life (0.55 per 1,000 prisoners) and those sentenced (0.83 per 1,000 prisoners). Offences of violence against the person carry significant risk of suicide. In 2020, 39 per cent of people who took their own life were prisoners either on remand or sentenced for these offences. Hanging is the most common method of self-inflicted death. In 2020 82 per cent of all suicides were by hanging or self-strangulation, with bedding the most commonly used ligature type, and windows the most commonly used ligature point (ONS, 2021).

Other factors include:

- **age** – younger men have higher rates of self-harm than older men, although men aged 30 plus who self-harm tend to do so in ways that result in more serious injury;
- **ethnicity** – self-harm rates are higher among white men;
- **educational background** – those lacking formal education are more likely to self-harm;
- **relationship status** – those who are single and/or had a recent relationship breakdown face increased risk;
- **accommodation** – there is increased risk to those who have no fixed abode outside prison;
- **a high number of disciplinary infractions** – this coincides with greater levels of self-harm (evidence suggests that prisoners who self-harm tend to act more aggressively towards themselves, other people and objects) and includes prisoners who are regularly transferred to Care and Separation Units, or so called 'Segregation Units';(Lohner and Konrad, 2006, 2007; Dixon-Gordon et al., 2012; Lanes, 2009).

As is the case outside of prison, the primary motive for self-harm in prison is emotional regulation (Dixon-Gordon et al., 2012). However, male prisoners who self-harm are often also motivated by 'instrumental' reasons, e.g. achieving an end goal or change in circumstances, achieving a transfer, getting material benefits or 'wanting help'. Adult men attempting suicide are most likely to be motivated by situational factors related directly to their imprisonment, but not specifically offence-related, such as 'depression', 'concern over children' or 'homesickness' (Snow, 2002). Prison can increase the sense of psychological entrapment and exacerbate a high external locus of control, ineffective coping and low resilience (Slade et al., 2014).

Common problems preceding self-harm in prison are not dissimilar to those experienced outside prison (see Table 1.8).

Table 1.8 Common problems preceding self-harm in prison

Previous trauma	Recent stressors
History of mental health problems, especially depression	Poor coping strategies
Low self esteem	Poor physical health
Anxiety	Substance misuse
Family problems	Change in circumstance, e.g. sentence
Difficulties or disputes with other prisoners/officers/ healthcare staff	Court appearances
Bullying and/or debt	Sexual problems

Those factors associated with repeated self-harm include:

- previous self-harm;
- personality disturbance;
- depression;
- alcohol or drug misuse;
- chronic psychosocial problems and behaviour disturbance;
- not feeling heard;
- not feeling helped.

Box 6: Occurrences that should prompt a re-assessment of risk

- When moving to a different part of the prison.
- When new people are involved in the person's care or significant people leave/ are away.
- Following a serious incident or an event that changes the context in which risk behaviours may occur.
- In anticipation of events known to increase risk, e.g. court appearances, sentencing, significant change etc.
- Before and after any significant change in treatment and/or the patient's management.
- After an incident of self-harm/suicide attempt or violent incident.
- Prior to and post discharge from the inpatient unit or CSU.

Staff-prisoner relationships and the impact on risk

Poor staff knowledge and attitudes can play a role in influencing self-harm. Evidence suggests negative attitudes from staff towards prisoners who self-harm are often based on what staff perceive as the motivation for, and purpose of, the behaviour. Staff who see it 'simply' as 'manipulative' or 'attention seeking' often then find it challenging to deal with (Snow, 2002). In many cases distinction is made between so called 'genuine' and 'non-genuine' self-harm. While 'genuine' self-harm may be associated with distress that can be attributed to actual events e.g. loss or major setback, 'non-genuine' self-harm or threat of self-harm can be perceived as a manipulative act, used by the prisoner to get something they otherwise wouldn't. This often evokes negative feelings in staff and adversely impacts on their individual and collective responses to the person (Ramluggun, 2013; Ireland and Quinn, 2007).

A prisoners' self-harm can be seen as further evidence of 'disruptive' behaviour, increasing the negative responses from some prison staff and, on occasions, 'trivialised' (Ireland and Quinn, 2007). This can be further complicated by some officers perceiving self-harm as a means for prisoners to influence or change their circumstances while healthcare staff view the self-harming behaviour as a sign of a prisoner's distress and/or inability to adapt to prison life (Ramluggun, 2013). Interdisciplinary conflict between staff, who think the other should deal with self-harm, can inhibit effective multidisciplinary working and put the individual prisoner at even greater risk (Ramluggan, 2013; Ireland and Quinn, 2007; Bennett and Dyson, 2014).

Assessing risk – prior to arrival in prison

Risk management for vulnerable prisoners starts prior to their arrival in prison. At the time of arrest there is an opportunity for police officers to detain the person under Section 136 and take them to a place of safety where they can be formally assessed by mental health professionals.

If a crime by someone who has a mental illness has been investigated, a decision can be made that a non-criminal justice disposal is appropriate, 'whether it is suitable to be charged by the police, or whether advice should be sought from the Crown Prosecution Service [CPS] on an appropriate charge'. The relevant information about that person's mental health should be obtained and included with the case file sent by the police to the CPS and court so that a properly informed decision can be made (HMIP, 2021). Police stations, custody suites and courts all have Liaison and Diversion (L&D) services usually staffed by mental health nurses employed by local NHS Trusts. It is their job to identify individuals who have mental health needs or other vulnerabilities when they first encounter the CJS as suspects, defendants or offenders. L&D staff carry out assessments to provide advice. This information is then shared in court and, where appropriate, people are given information about agencies that can support the person and help them be diverted from the CJS and referred to an appropriate health or social care service or appropriate setting.

However, 'A Joint Thematic Inspection of the Criminal Justice Journey for Individuals with Mental Health Need and Disorders' (HMIP, 2021) identified significant problems at every stage of the person's journey, from communication, access to services and transfer into hospital.

Those individuals known to pose a higher risk of harm to others, including violent and sexual offenders, come under The Multi-Agency Public Protection Arrangements (MAPPA), introduced in 2001. MAPPA is aimed at improving inter-agency collaboration. Organised at the police force area, probation, police and prison services come together to form the MAPPA Responsible Authority area. Other agencies, such as the NHS or local authorities, have a duty to cooperate with MAPPA. The task of the MAPPA group is to work together locally to identify, assess and manage the heightened risk. This is done in part through Management of Sexual or Violent Offenders (MOSOVO) teams and officers. Multi-agency risk assessment conferences (MARAC) address the highest risk domestic abuse offenders. In all these processes mental health services are either directly involved or are used as a critical pathway when applicable to the offender being considered. This structured, multi-agency approach has been associated with 'significant falls in re-offending' (HM Inspectorate of Probation, 2021).

Thus, by the time a vulnerable prisoner arrives in prison, there have been several occasions when their mental health and risk should have been assessed, and for them to be either diverted into mental health services such as an appropriate psychiatric unit, or reports written to accompany the prisoner identifying existing mental health issues as well as potential or actual risk.

Assessing risk – reception screening

This does not mean that every person with significant mental health problems who might pose a risk to themselves and/or others has been identified and a risk management plan put in place. A robust screening process is required for every person entering prison.

It involves prison staff asking about the person's level of risk for sharing a cell, a very brief overview of any drug or alcohol misuse, any violence or involvement with extremist groups or extremist ideas in the person's past and a cursory assessment of risk to self and any mental health issues. A more detailed assessment of the person's healthcare needs is made by a nurse, with a template for assessing the person's physical health, mental health, drug and alcohol use, any self-harm and suicidal thoughts. However, while this takes a minimum of 10–20 minutes to complete properly (and longer for someone with complex health problems and/or risks), some prisons will have upwards of a dozen prisoners arrive together, almost always after 5pm, with the nurse only having 2–3 hours in which to see each one of them.

As a result, the reception screening is complicated in practice by the time of arrival of prisoners, the numbers arriving and the limited time in which to carry out the screening. In addition, the prisoner may be tired, hungry and thirsty, stressed by the experience of their arrest or court appearance or simply reluctant to tell their story again. The nurse or clinician (though, ideally, it should be a registered nurse) undertaking the screening has to be aware the person may be wary of revealing any vulnerabilities. This could be a very practical issue, because the environment is not particularly private and there is a possibility of other prisoners overhearing the conversation, or the person may have other reasons, e.g. feelings of shame, or being unsure how the information they provide will be used if they are new to prison.

The better the relationship between the nurse with officers in the reception area – and the more aware they are of the nurse's role and responsibilities – the more opportunities to have the support of discipline staff and to get sufficient time without interruption for prisoners who need it.

The process is further complicated by factors that might motivate prisoners to fabricate their answers. Mental health problems and/or the risk of self-harm or suicide may garner more time from clinicians, medication or even time in an inpatient unit within the prison, away from what can be seen as the stressful environment of the main prison. Having mental health problems could lead to someone being placed in a single cell, often a prized location within the prison environment, though risk to self usually means the person would be expected to share as this is viewed as safer. Conversely, a prisoner convincing staff that they pose a threat of violence to others means the person is likely to be placed in a single cell, even if other sanctions may be imposed.

Reception screening, therefore, requires the skills of building a rapport and rapid assessment more akin to a triage. Where the reception staff have access to the same electronic records system as L&D services and local Trusts, accessing and making use of any such records is an essential part of the screening. However, as with every other assessment process described in the *Pocket Guide*, much will be down to what the assessor is looking for and what they are able to identify themselves.

Any template-based interview works most effectively when the clinician is familiar with the questions and can create, from them, a conversation about the person's health. Again, the interview utilises all the techniques highlighted in earlier sections of *The Pocket Guide,* including keeping the questions brief and simple, making eye contact, active listening, clinical curiosity and funnelling in on important issues. NICE Guidelines (2016) simply note the clinician must enter all answers into the patient's record, plus health-related observations 'including those about behaviour and mental state (including eye contact, body language, rapid, slow or strange speech, poor hygiene, strange thoughts) and "details of any action taken"'.

Looking at the computer screen to read the questions as they're written and writing in the answers as the interview progresses clearly breaks up the flow of the conversation – with the risk of turning it into a question and answer session which can then come across as a tick box exercise and potentially alienating. It may limit the opportunities to get any meaningful information, especially if the questions are asked as they are on many of the templates, with an abrupt shift to mental health from physical health. With entries that only require a closed question, such as, 'have you ever seen a psychiatrist?' and 'have you ever self-harmed or attempted suicide?', it is easy to see how clinicians can 'lose' the prisoner and miss out on important information.

The importance of the reception screening is emphasised by harsh statistics:

- In 2020, 14 (21 per cent) of all self-inflicted deaths occurred within the first 30 days of custody.
- Seven (50 per cent) occurred within the first week.
- In 2020 when including prisoners who have moved, 23 (34 per cent) self-inflicted deaths occurred within the first 30 days in the current prison.
- Ten (43 per cent) occurred within the first week.

In some prisons a mental health nurse and substance misuse clinician will be present and can immediately address any issues within their area of expertise. In all cases, if there are any concerns about the person's health the reception clinician is expected to refer the patient to the appropriate service. If the concern is about the risk of self-harm or suicide, an ACCT is opened (see below).

Assessing risk – secondary screening

Within a week of the person arriving in prison, a secondary screen is required by the healthcare team (NICE, 2016). This is often classed as a health and wellbeing assessment, taking a rounded approach to finding out more about the person, their current and past health and social issues, as well as how they are likely to adjust to being in prison. This explores all areas of the person's physical and mental health and any substance misuse issues, as well as historical and current risk. Again, there are challenges about time but this *full assessment* needs to be conducted with the rigour and depth required to create an in depth understanding of the person's health, wellbeing and risk while in prison.

The ACCT process

The Assessment, Care in Custody and Teamwork (ACCT), first developed in 2005 and revised in 2021, is the care planning and case management system for prisoners identified as being at risk of self-harm or suicide, with defined actions designed to reduce the risk. It sets out a timescale and process of assessing the risk and then for scheduled reviews. With the responsibility for the process held and led by the prison, officers of a designated seniority, specially trained in risk assessment, must undertake the initial assessment and subsequent reviews. In 2019, the number of people put on an ACCT was 27,389 compared to 17,314 in 2010, an increase of 60 per cent (Allison and McIntyre, 2021).

Anyone in a prison can open an ACCT at any time, including in reception. In some establishments, certain factors which heighten the risk of suicide will automatically trigger an ACCT assessment, e.g. being convicted of homicide or receiving a long sentence.

The criteria are relatively flexible. It may follow an actual episode of self-harm or suicide attempt. The prisoner may have expressed concern about their safety or risk may have been identified during a routine contact by a member of staff. The ACCT remains active until the person is no longer considered to be at risk, then remains in a post-closure state for a week and can be re-opened if further concerns about the person's safety arise.

Nonetheless, despite such an organised, structured process, the assessment and management of risk still comes down to the ability of the assessor to engage the person and combine their actuarial knowledge of clinical risk factors with the information they gain about the person to reach a structured professional judgement. The same risks of using the helpful (and evidence based) prompts in a way that renders it a 'tick box exercise' exist, just as they do with the reception screening. Other potential problems are that the multi professional approach it is designed to promote, so successful with MAPPA offenders, doesn't happen, or that there is no consistency, with different reviewers stepping in or clinicians who don't know the prisoner present but not actively participating. That 24 out of 92 people who took their life in 2018 while in custody were on an ACCT underlines the importance of adhering to a rigorous process and avoiding the pitfalls outlined above.

Instrumental threats of self-harm and 'malingering'

There can be times in an assessment when the clinician asks themselves, 'do I really believe this?' It might be that the person is denying or minimising the risk or the opposite – talking about serious self-harm and even suicide, but in such a way that the clinician does not think the person will actually carry out the act.

In a prison setting, it is not unknown to hear a prisoner state, "If I don't get a vape I'm going to cut up." For 'vape', one can substitute TV, single cell or any number of things the person wants at that time. This is the type of instrumental self-harm referred to in the section on 'staff-prisoner relationships and the impact on risk' (page 69), which is often characterised as 'non genuine'. In fact, the motives are likely to be complex and still merit the same assessment process as any other type of risk. Consideration of why this has suddenly become an issue at this time is highly relevant. It's just as necessary to explore what the person is thinking, how they feel and how this is impacting on their behaviour, validating their perception if not agreeing or colluding with the behaviour, as it would be in any assessment.

What will be different is the response from the clinician and prison staff. If there is a valid reason for the person not to have what it is they are seeking, this needs to be communicated clearly, the context explained and the decision applied consistently, with a plan put in place to reasonably support the person while maintaining the rules of the institution and clear boundaries. If there is any perceived inequity or unfairness, this needs to be addressed. For officers, particularly, this is a key factor in their safe management of the prisoners in their charge and the prison itself. Healthcare staff need to support this while being available for the prisoner if there are health related factors or as part of the person's ACCT review. Beyond any risk management plan, however, is a deeper issue to be explored: why does the person feel impelled to behave in this way? Why threaten harm to themselves to obtain something they could presumably achieve through other, simpler means, e.g. following the rules of the prison, seeking help from staff? This is the behaviour often labelled 'manipulation' or 'attention seeking' but, looking back to the analysis by Linehan (2015) on page 46, we are reminded that these behaviours lack the subtlety and deviousness associated with the skills required for manipulation but are often desperate, naive, and inappropriate attempts by the person to have their emotional needs met, to find validation, approval, praise or care. It is this that needs to be addressed, in addition to maintaining boundaries and managing risk.

If the person is suspected of fabricating physical illness, it is easier to assess this in that it's possible to perform diagnostic tests e.g. bloods, ECG, X rays or whatever else is needed. However, some of these may involve being seen in an outside hospital and necessitate assessing the potential risks of the person being taken from the prison for further tests. If the concern is about substance misuse, an immediate urinalysis can be undertaken to identify the presence of drugs like opiates, cocaine, benzodiazepines and cannabis etc, while toxicology tests can be carried out on blood samples.

There is a lot of discussion in the *Pocket Guide* about people minimising their thoughts about harming themselves or others or mental health symptoms, and what might lie behind this. Many clinicians – especially those working in prisons – will be familiar with the opposite: instances when they think a person is exaggerating or even fabricating their symptoms. Perhaps it will relate to an account of auditory or visual hallucinations, depression or anxiety. It is often referred to as 'malingering'. This is *not* factitious disorder, a serious mental health disorder which involves people deliberately producing symptoms of an illness for the purpose of receiving care and attention in a medical setting. In factitious disorders, the symptoms aren't 'instrumental' or have the intention of helping the person get practical benefits. The gain is believed to be psychological.

The *Diagnostic and Statistical Manual of Mental Disorders* (2013) describes malingering as the intentional production of false or grossly exaggerated physical or psychological problems. It is usually associated with an attempt to 'gain external benefits such as avoiding work or responsibility, seeking drugs, avoiding trial (law), seeking attention, avoiding military service, leave from school, paid leave from a job, among others' (Alozai and McPherson, 2023.

But how does a clinician conclude the person in front of them is malingering? For example, anxiety is a subjective experience, much as physical pain is now recognised to be. Equally, it is possible to subjectively 'feel' depressed without having poor sleep, loss of appetite or other symptoms of clinical depression. People may describe themselves as extremely anxious or depressed despite others finding this difficult to understand or there being lots of objective 'evidence' that seems to contradict this. Determining whether or not someone is having a psychotic experience, i.e. having lost contact with reality, is another matter. Well documented problems with diagnosis aside (see, for example, Aboraya et al., 2006), there may be understandable reasons a prisoner would exaggerate or fabricate symptoms. They may believe they will be admitted to the healthcare unit or even transferred from prison to hospital, be prescribed medication they want, get a single cell or gain some other advantage.

To those having to assess them or provide care for them, this may be infuriating but, for the person, all of these things may be a means of ultimately feeling safe, whatever superficial motivation they or others attribute to them. It can also be interpreted as a form of non-engaging engagement, i.e. while the person is engaging with healthcare staff, it is not about their actual 'problem' – indeed, may even distract from it – and encourages an avenue of enquiry and activity that will not prove helpful, as well as potentially creating a very difficult relationship between staff and the patient. It's also possible patients who have experienced psychotic symptoms may, at another stage of their stay in prison, fabricate different symptoms or report a recurrence in symptoms which is not genuine.

It is, therefore, very complex. However, there are possible indicators of 'malingered' psychosis from the outset. The person may well be calling attention to the 'illness', wanting to talk about it at length and overacting the symptoms they ascribe to their psychosis. They may have difficulties maintaining consistency in their overall presentation, with noticeable contradictions to their account. There may have been a sudden onset and equally sudden termination of delusions and/or other symptoms. Although there is reference in different sections of the *Pocket Guide* to clinical presentations where a lack of congruence is a feature, in the case of malingering, this is often seen between the person's description of extremely disturbing experiences and an affect that doesn't reflect that level of disturbance. Part of the individual's presentation may include attempts to intimidate clinicians and much of the literature cites potential risk to clinicians undertaking the assessment; see, for example, Alozai and McPherson (2023). As the interview progresses, their responses may also include a number of 'I don't knows' as, the more the clinician probes, the person's knowledge of symptoms or what to say may run dry (Resnick, 2015). Finally, malingerers frequently show poor compliance with treatment and stop complaining about the assumed illness only after gaining the external benefit.

The depth and detail of the assessment will almost certainly be important in helping the clinician understand the person's presentation and mental state – of course, including reasons the person may be malingering if that is thought to be the case.

The assessment will have to focus on issues identified above, e.g.:

- congruence between affect and descriptions of distressing/disturbing experiences;
- consistency in the person's story;
- adherence to the assessment process;
- being aware of any exaggeration or dramatic presentation of symptoms.

Open ended questions will be difficult to answer if the person is malingering while the clinician needs to be careful to avoid leading questions that provide the answer within the framework of the question, e.g. "How long have you been hearing voices?" It would be better to say "Tell me about your experiences," followed by "Say a bit more about that," etc.

There are specific assessment tools that can be used, such as the Miller Forensic Assessment of Symptoms Test or Structured Interview of Reported Symptoms, which can be useful in arriving at a decision. Ultimately, the same issues about understanding the nature of any risk and putting in place a robust plan to manage any actual or potential risk take precedence. Part of this is to understand why the person might be malingering and how they will react if they do not achieve the goals that motivated them in the first place.

Structural changes that can increase patient safety

The risk assessment and management process inside prisons is complicated by very specific, prison-related, factors. These need to be addressed both by the prison and healthcare provider, including:

- Providing specialist training to all clinicians working within this environment to equip them with the knowledge and skills required, particularly focusing on:
  - mental health awareness;
  - understanding personality disorder;

- risk assessment of suicide and self-harm;
- risk assessment of violence;
- reception screening;
- advanced communication skills.

- Allocating sufficient staff to reception screening and secondary screening to enable the practitioner to fully complete the screenings and give the prisoner the time needed.
- Establishing systems for the organisation of ACCTs, providing consistent attendance by the reviewer and enabling healthcare teams to prepare for the review and have the same, suitably skilled, practitioner attend the reviews.
- Prioritising safe and confidential spaces within the prison for clinicians to conduct risk assessments and subsequent treatment sessions.
- Setting up forums that support clinicians in their work, providing reflective practice and clinical supervision, as well as complex case discussions (though these may be viewed as being accommodated by weekly Safety and Intervention Meetings [SIM] and Challenge Support Intervention Plan [CSIP] meetings, these are run by the prison, are multi professional and not many healthcare practitioners will attend).
- Using a risk management system such as zoning[xvi] to assist them in prioritising and managing the work of their patient group.
- The use of structured sessions throughout the day to support staff, help them prioritise their work that day and provide feedback on the highest risk patients. These might include planning sessions in the morning and a lunchtime 'huddle' when staff can report back and receive support if needed, with a final evaluation meeting in the evening for staff to discuss their day and begin the planning process for the next day.

Violence in prison

The rate of violent assaults in prison more than doubled between 2014 and 2018. It's probable that better reporting and recording accounts for some of this but it was an extraordinary development, with 31,025 assaults (29,768 perpetrated in male establishments) from March 2017–2018, including 9,003 assaults on staff in 2018, more than double that in 2015. Both were record highs and occurred in the context of a loss of 3,789 officers between 2010 and 2018, most with many years of experience. Indeed, 70,000 years of officer experience was lost with those who quit the service during that period (Savage, 2018).

Recognising that there is a wider context and a range of environmental and organisational circumstances affecting violence within prisons, two models have been identified to aid an understanding of the phenomenon (see Box 7).

Box 7:   Models of violence in prison

The deprivation model

- Prison environment and loss of freedom cause deep psychological trauma.
- For psychological self-preservation prisoners create a deviant prison subculture that promotes violence. (Sykes, 1958; Farrington and Nuttall, 1980; Wortley, 2003).

The importation model

Prisoners bring into the institution:

- their histories;
- personal attitudes;
- social networks, including links to criminal groups, gangs etc (Cao, Zhao and Vandine, 1997; Harer and Steffensmeier, 1996).

Another way of understanding violence in prison is the KGH Pathway to Violence (Sinai et al., 2017). Many of the perpetrators of violence, even relatively minor violence, will have gone through the same process of:

- a cognitive opening;
- triggering events;
- grievance;
- ideation/fantasy;
- planning;
- preparation;
- implementation.

Factors influencing violence in prison

Around 85–90 per cent of violent offenders are male, with the majority of perpetrators aged 16–29. They have usually experienced a lack of discipline or arbitrary and inconsistent discipline at home and had low levels of parental supervision.

External, structural and situational factors that will impact on violence in the institution will include:

- prison architecture and design;
- levels of security;
- management practices, e.g. staffing models, staff skills and training, prison culture and management style;
- outside environmental influences, e.g. political pressures on prison administrators, racial tensions.

Factors influencing violence in individual prisoners

- Previous aggressive or violent behavior.
- Being the victim of physical abuse and/or sexual abuse.
- Exposure to violence in the home and/or community.
- Genetic (family heredity) factors.
- Unstable self-esteem.
- Combination of stressful family socioeconomic factors (poverty, severe deprivation, marital breakup, poor parenting, unemployment, loss of support from extended family).
- Brain damage from head trauma, e.g. injury, infection, etc.

- Substance misuse.
- Lack of sleep.
- Lack of guilt that is linked to likelihood of offending.
- Attitudinal factors such as 'positive attitudes to problem behaviour' (Beyers et al., 2001).
- Associating with delinquent peers and having previously offended.

It is perhaps little surprise that victims of violence are almost a mirror image of its perpetrators. They are most likely to be young men, often experiencing many of the same familial problems as the offenders. Their personality characteristics include many similar to those of offenders as well.

Assessing risk – forensic units

Forensic mental health has been defined as: 'an area of specialisation that, in the criminal sphere, involves the assessment and *treatment* of those who are both mentally disordered and whose behaviour has led, or could lead, to offending' (Mullen, 2000). Harty and Walsh (2018) describe forensic patients as having 'mental disorders which make them a potential risk to others, and who may have offended or be judged likely to offend'. Forensic services are tiered, being identified as 'low', 'medium' and 'high'. These have been defined by NHS England (2021) as:

- 'High Secure services provide care and treatment to those adults who present a **grave and immediate risk to the public** and who must not be able to escape from hospital.
- Medium secure services provide care and treatment to those adults who present a **serious** risk of harm to others and whose escape from hospital must be prevented.
- Low secure services provide care and treatment who present a **significant** risk of harm to others and whose escape from hospital must be impeded'.

NHS forensic services will also have outreach and liaison services to provide care and treatment for those in the community. People can be admitted to forensic units from the courts, non-secure psychiatric units and, of course, prison. They will be detained under the Mental Health Act, thus having no clear idea when their period of detention will end (prison sentences are of a determinate period, although the person may be subject to release on licence, which means they can be recalled if they re-offend). This creates uncertainty and can lead to resentment towards the clinical team if the patient attributes blame to them for being detained. It may also lead to the patient trying to withhold information about risk, among other things, for fear it will prolong their period of detention. Markham (2020) notes:

> At times, the patient may not accept the clinician's or care team's views of his or her risk. In that case, the patient's trust in the clinician and treatment will decrease; cognitive distortions may develop leading to problems in compliance. Hence … portions of the risk assessment may need to be kept confidential, especially in cases where the patient needs to be monitored in the long term to prevent harm to others.

Even though the context is obviously different, the principles of risk assessment and risk management, as outlined in earlier sections of *The Pocket Guide*, are applicable, i.e. identifying potential or actual risk, the likelihood of risk behaviours occurring and

Table 1.9 Structured clinical assessment of violence risk (adapted from Maden, 2007)

Stage 1	Gathering information, using patient records, court reports etc, interviewing the person and speaking with relatives/carers and other informants
Stage 2	Standardised assessment of static and dynamic risk factors
Stage 3	Consideration of idiosyncratic risk factors
Stage 4	Description of risk to others, including the specific nature of the risk, e.g. physical assault, potential victims, factors that increase/decrease the risk
Stage 5	Risk management plan, including contingency plans
Stage 6	Prioritising actions of the team and who will do what

developing a plan to minimise harmful outcomes and maximise beneficial outcomes, and do not need to be repeated here. However, it is important to consider what is different about doing this work in a forensic environment. Forensic patients may pose a serious risk to themselves, and forensic risk assessment primarily focuses on the potential for risk to others, but Monahan et al. (2001) argue that clinicians' unaided assessments of risk to others or dangerousness are barely better than chance. There is also the risk of potential outcomes such as 'false positives' and 'false negatives'. False positives occur when assessors are overly cautious or overestimate the risk, resulting in mistakenly concluding the risk is more significant and serious than it actually is. False negatives occur when the assessor underestimates the level of risk.

The structure and content of the assessment format is, essentially, no different to that of a mental health assessment incorporating the assessment of risk. One element that is different is the attention to detail in a forensic risk assessment and the sharp focus on risk to others. Different methods are used. The structured clinical assessment of violence risk combines standardised and clinical methods (Maden, 2007). It is widely used and assists clinicians in identifying key information about the patient to collect and then arrive at their own decisions about what to do with it in specific stages (see Table 1.9).

A commonly used tool for structured clinical assessment of violence risk – though there are a number of others – is the HCR-20. This is a 20 item structured framework for the assessment of violence risk intended for use with civil psychiatric, community, forensic and criminal justice populations. It's broken up into different sections:

- historical items;
- clinical items;
- risk management items.

Each item is scored as:

- definitely present (scores 2);
- probably or partially present (scores 1);
- absent (scores 0).

Although the items are carefully defined, there is still an element of subjective judgement in some. There is also a risk – as is the case in all structured clinical assessments – of focusing so intently on risk that the person is 'lost', their real needs and even why they may pose the risks to others identified overlooked. Building a relationship with the patient, then, which supports openness and transparency within an ethical framework, that can safely contain strongly differing views between the clinical team and the patient, but where clinicians are equipped with advanced engagement and motivational interviewing skills – recognising that many patients are, at best, reluctant participants in the treatment process – are all required in a forensic environment. Parallel to the use of tools to assess risk, using tools such as the Structured Assessment of Protective Factors (De Vogel et al., 2012) can be useful in creating a balance and overcoming potential biases that skew the judgement of risk.

Developing a common language for assessing and communicating risk

There are significant differences in the various types of risk assessment you might undertake, for example:

- a triage assessment for the purpose of referring to a specialist team or deciding on a care pathway;
- an initial assessment of risk to determine a risk management plan;
- a re-assessment of someone where risk has previously been established.

There are inherent problems in using terminology such as 'short, medium or long term' etc, as these are subjective and open to interpretation. Ideally, it is better to think of risk in terms of whether it is:

- immediate i.e. likely to happen now;
- in the future, in which case, what would need to happen to make it more likely the risk would become imminent?

Again, rather than describe risk in vague language such as 'low', 'medium' or 'high' (when, for instance does 'short term' become 'medium term' and when does that end?), it is more useful to describe risk in terms of risk factors. These can be as follows.

Static

These are fixed, historical factors, e.g. gender, family history of suicide, violence, previous hospital admissions, previous risk incidents. They are not anything that can be changed, therefore not something to 'treat' and do not provide an authoritative guide to risk or whether or not it has changed. However, they can provide a baseline or guide to how the person may behave in certain circumstances, e.g. if they are making threats are they likely to carry them out? Have there been acts of violence in the past? What were the circumstances? Was it linked to substance misuse, increased stress, psychotic symptoms or feeling threatened? As such, you cannot afford to ignore static factors.

Stable

Long term factors, e.g. diagnosis of personality disorder or mental health problems. Of course, in many cases, diagnosis can change, either as the person becomes better known to clinicians or new information comes to light through the assessment and treatment process. It then becomes important to re-evaluate issues of risk. These factors are not liable to fluctuate in a short space of time or be as vulnerable to change as dynamic factors.

Dynamic

These are present but fluctuate in duration and intensity, e.g. hopelessness, stress, treatment adherence, substance misuse or the opportunity to act in a dangerous way. It is important to consider these *measurable* factors in terms of treatment precisely because it is these that are susceptible to treatment and risk management interventions. Reducing these risk factors and their impact on the person and their behaviour is important.

Future

This involves trying to anticipate potential risk(s), particularly given any knowledge of past risks.

The nature of different elements of the person's risk profile can then be identified more clearly and precisely, allowing the clinician to think about the focus of immediate and longer term risk management plans. For example:

> William has a history of attempting to end his life by paracetamol overdose in the context of a relationship breakup (*static risk factor*). Last night, he took 18 paracetamol 500mg tablets with the intention of killing himself after his partner left him. He has been clinically depressed for several months (*Stable risk factor*) but is now feeling hopeless, can see no future for himself and has disengaged from services (*Dynamic risk factors*). He currently still has plans to kill himself, using tablets, self poisoning or hanging, given the opportunity (*future risk factor*).

However, there may still be a desire to use terminology such as 'low', 'medium' and 'high' risk (as may be the case, for instance, in non mental health clinicians who have conducted a brief assessment (or perhaps a triage in an Emergency Department) and want to communicate the urgency of the referral to the mental health team taking the referral). It is then essential that there are written definitions that clinicians can refer to and the understanding of which is widely shared and acknowledged (see Tables 1.10, 1.11 and 1.12 below).

As stated earlier, one of the significant advantages of using recognised screening or risk assessment tools is that they provide a common language.

Table 1.10 An example of Definitions of Risk Levels – Low Risk (adapted from Hart, Colley and Harrison, 2009)

LOW RISK	ACTION REQUIRED
A patient who has been assessed will be deemed to be 'low risk' if: • there are no significant mental health problems present; • there may have been some risk behaviours present, e.g. excessive drinking or substance abuse, superficial cutting, but these have not led to significant physical harm and there are sufficient protective factors to suggest the patient is unlikely to deteriorate; • they have no current plans to harm themselves and/or others; • they are not vulnerable to self neglect or exploitation by others; • it is not thought there will be a deterioration in their mental state or situation that would significantly increase the levels of risk in the foreseeable future.	• No immediate action is required to address issues related to the patient's risk factors. • It may be helpful to look at alternative coping strategies with the patient. • The patient may benefit from health education/advice about potentially harmful behaviours, e.g. drinking and/or substance abuse, poor sleep etc. • The patient may be referred to primary care or voluntary sector services, where potentially harmful behaviours can be addressed with the patient if they wish, but this would be on a routine basis.

Table 1.11 An example of Definitions of Risk Levels – Medium Risk (adapted from Hart, Colley and Harrison, 2009)

MEDIUM RISK	ACTION REQUIRED
• **A patient who has been assessed will be deemed to be 'medium risk' if one or more of the following are present:** • mental health problems impacting on their overall functioning; • they have self injured or harmed others but the injuries sustained did not require serious medical treatment; • they have plans to harm themselves and/or others but these are not immediate; • while the risk factors are not current, there is a probability they will become present in the absence of care and treatment; • they would be vulnerable to serious self neglect or exploitation by others in foreseeable circumstances; • there is the possibility of deterioration in their mental state or situation that may significantly increase the levels of risk if they are not in receipt of mental health care and treatment.	• All areas of risk (actual and potential) must be clearly identified, with exacerbating and protective factors. • Attempts should be made to engage the patient in active treatment to address risk factors, beginning with agreeing a risk management plan, incorporating who will be doing what to help the patient remain safe. • Alternative coping strategies should be explored and expanded upon if necessary. • If a risk management plan is agreed, this should be fully documented and communicated to all clinicians (and others) who may have a role in assisting the patient in remaining safe. • If the patient doesn't wish to engage in any risk management, nor commit themselves to remain safe, a capacity assessment should be carried out. Decisions are required about how best to assist the patient, including whether or not a more restrictive environment is required and if there is a need for a Mental Health Act assessment. • If the risk is potential rather than actual, or assessed as not requiring immediate intervention, it should be made clear to the person how to contact services, particularly crisis services, and further contact again offered by the clinicians assessing the person. • All relevant clinicians and agencies, e.g. GP, should be informed of the risk assessment and outcome and advised about what action to take if they are contacted and the situation has deteriorated. • If the risk is actual and current, i.e. the patient is doing something dangerous and unwilling to engage, the risk should be re-defined as 'high' and the response should be as below.

Table 1.12 An example of Definitions of Risk Levels – High Risk (adapted from Hart, Colley and Harrison, 2009)

HIGH RISK	ACTION REQUIRED
A patient who has been assessed will be deemed to be 'high risk' if one or more of the following are present: • significant mental health problems are present and impairing the person's functioning; • they have plans to seriously harm or kill themselves and/or seriously harm others and these are immediate; • there are significant risk factors which are current; • there is a likelihood these will increase in the absence of mental health care and treatment; • they could be vulnerable to serious self neglect or exploitation by others; • there is a likelihood of deterioration in the person's mental state or situation that will significantly increase the levels of risk if they are not in receipt of mental health care and treatment.	• All areas of risk (actual and potential) must be clearly identified, including exacerbating and protective factors. • Attempts should be made to immediately engage the patient in active treatment to address risk factors. • A risk management plan, incorporating who will be doing what to help the patient remain safe addressing all immediate and ongoing risk factors, including a treatment and care package, should be communicated to all clinicians and agencies involved as well as any other relevant parties. • If the patient is not willing or able to engage, a safety care plan should be imposed. A more restrictive setting should be considered and a Mental Health Act assessment arranged for the earliest possible time. • If the patient is in an inpatient unit or Emergency Department, they should not be allowed to leave until the Mental Health Act assessment is complete.

NB: Patients newly admitted to a mental health service and not fully assessed should be regarded as medium to high risk in terms of risk management.

These criteria also confirm that the lack of a diagnosed mental disorder should not preclude a risk management plan being put in place and implemented.

Key clinical tip – developing common language

Terminology such as 'high', 'low', short, medium and long term can be highly subjective and lead to misunderstanding and errors. Wherever they have to be used, a team should have clear, written definitions of what they mean and ensure clinicians using them understand their meaning.

Notes

   i This involved interviewing 7,500 people aged 16 and over across all communities in the UK to obtain a large representative sample. It's carried out every seven years. The fieldwork was carried out in 2014 and 2015.

  ii See Jonny Benjamin and Neil Laybourn talking together on YouTube: https://www.youtube.com/watch?v=n2BIfTXfcCs.

 iii More than 160,000 Americans died in 2017 from suicide (47,173), drug overdose (70,237) and alcohol related liver disease (44,478).

 iv As worrying as these figures are, the latest statistics from the World Health Organisation show the highest number of suicides in the 25–34 age group, at 23.84 per 100,000 population when male and female numbers are combined. Male suicides in this age group are 37.45 per 100,000 population.

  v Economically inactive, i.e. out of work, not actively looking for work, not waiting to start a job, not in full-time education.

 vi Job insecurity is defined as 'those who are underemployed, report volatile pay or hours, are in non permanent work (where this isn't their choice), or are in low paid self employment'. Those meeting more than one of these measures were not double counted in a survey of 2021 employees (Living Wage Foundation, 2022).

 vii All figures for suicide indicate the year the suicide was registered, not necessarily the year in which the death occurred.

viii Figures were unavailable for Pakistani women.

 ix Note: the Office for National Statistics don't use the same categories as were identified by the APMS team.

  x It is of interest that there are some similarities between the Integrated Motivational – Volitional Model of Suicidal Behaviour and the The KGH Pathway to Violence Model (see page 59), suggesting that there is a similar process that takes people down the psychological pathway to both violence and suicide. There are examples of interviews with perpetrators of homicide which highlight this and how the process that might lead to suicide can alter to one of homicide. One such case was Will Cornick, convicted of the murder of his teacher, Ann McGuire. Cornick 'told a psychiatrist that he decided four days before the killing, on a Thursday, that he was going to murder Maguire rather than kill himself,' adding, "I did not have a choice. It was kill her or suicide." (Pidd, 2014.) Darren Osbourne, convicted of the murder of Makram Ali after deliberately driving a van at a crowd of Muslims outside Finsbury Park Mosque in 2017, was noted to have previously expressed suicidal ideas.

 xi For statistics around suicide and prisoners, see Risk factors specific to prison (p. 128)

 xii This is people under the care of a mental health team, either in an inpatient or community setting.

xiii All figures taken from the Office for National Statistics website (www.ons.gov.uk) unless otherwise stated.

xiv See page 87 for more information on reception screening.

 xv These are the prison-based equivalent of community mental health teams. Except that, instead of going out into the community to see patients, they 'reach in' to the prison to see their patients on the house block or wing where the patient resides.

xvi A 'traffic light' system for categorising risk levels, e.g. red for the most at risk, amber for the next highest level and green for those posing the least risk. With clear definitions of the risk criteria for different categories there are also standards for the team's interventions, e.g. someone in the red zone being seen every day. A similar approach can be made to categorising new referrals, e.g. crisis, urgent and routine, with standards for how quickly the person will be seen, reviewed by the team and action taken in initiating interventions, if required.

References and selected bibliography

Aboraya, A., Rankin€, E., France, C., El-Missiry, A. and John, C. (2006) The Reliability of Psychiatric Diagnosis Revisited: The Clinician's Guide to Improve the Reliability of Psychiatric Diagnosis. *Psychiatry*, 3(1), January, 41–50.

Abrutyn, S., Mueller, A.S. and Osbourne, M. (2019) Rekeying Cultural Scripts for Youth Suicide: How Social Networks Facilitate Suicide Diffusion and Suicide Clusters Following Exposure to Suicide. *Society and Mental Health*, 10(2).

Addictions UK (2022) Alcoholism and Suicide. www.addictions.uk.

Alerdice, J., Morgan, J., Antoniou, J., Bolton, J., Brown, T., Cassidy, C., Daw, R., Dennis, M., Edgar, K., Ferns, J, Fisher, A., Hawton, K., Kamerling, V., O'Connor, R., Palmer, L., Trainor, G. and Wilson, M. (2010) *Self-harm, suicide and risk: helping people who self-harm*. London: Royal College of Psychiatry.

Allison, E. and McIntyre, N. (2021) Number of prisoners in England and Wales on suicide watch rises steeply. *The Guardian*, 10 February.

Allnutt, S., O'Driscoll, C., Ogloff, J.R.P., Daffern, M. and Adams, J. (2010) *Clinical Risk Assessment & Management: A Practical Manual for Mental Health Clinicians*. Sydney, NSW; Justice Health.

Alozai, U.U. and McPherson, P.K. (2023) Malingering. In: StatPearls [Internet]. Treasure Island (FL): StatPearls Publishing. PMID: 29939614.

Alvarez, A. (2002) *The Savage God*. London: Bloomsbury.

American Psychiatric Association (2013) *Diagnostic and Statistical Manual of Mental Disorders*, 5th ed. Arlington, VA, USA: American Psychiatric Association.

Appleby, L., Shaw, J., Kapur, N., Windfuhr, K., Ashton, A., Swinson, N. and While, D. (2006) *Avoidable Deaths: Five Year Report by the National Confidential Inquiry into Suicide and Homicide By People with Mental Illness*. Manchester: University of Manchester.

Appleby, L., Kapur, N., Shaw, J., Turnball, P., Hunt, I.M., Ibrahim, S., Bojanic, L., Graney, J., Baird, A., Rodway, C., Tham, S.G., and Burns, J. (2022) The National Confidential Inquiry into Suicide and Safety in Mental Health. Annual Report: UK patient and general population data, 2009–2019, and real time surveillance data. University of Manchester.

Atkinson, A. and Aldrick, P. (2022) UK Real Wages Post Their Biggest Drop in Two Decades. Bloomberg.com, accessed 27 August 2022.

Baker, C. (2021) *Suicide: summary of statistics*. House of Commons Library.

Barnes, M.C., Gunnell, D., Davies, R., Hawton, K., Kapur, N., Potokar, J. and Donovan, J.L. (2016) Understanding vulnerability to self-harm in times of economic hardship and austerity: a qualitative study. *BMJ Open*, 6, e010131. DOI: 10.1136/bmjopen-2015–010131.

Bebbington, P., Cooper, C., Minot, S., Brugha, T.S., Jenkins, R., Meltzer, H., Dennis, M. (2009) Suicide attempts, gender and sexual abuse: Data from the British psychiatric morbidity survey 2000. *American Journal of Psychiatry*, 166, 1135–1140.

Bebbington, P., Jakobowitz, S., McKenzie, N., Killaspy, H., Iveson, R., Duffield, G. and Kerr, M. (2017) Assessing needs for psychiatric treatment in prisoners: 1. Prevalence of disorder. *Social Psychiatry and Psychiatric Epidemiology*, 52(2), February, 221–229. DOI: 10.1007/s00127-016-1311–7. Epub 2016 Nov 22. PMID: 27878322; PMCID: PMC5329095.

Bennett, L. and Dyson, J. (2014) Deliberate self-harm among adults in prisons. *Mental Health Practice*, 18(1), 14–20.

Bergen, H., Hawton, K., Waters, K., Cooper, J. and Kapur, N. (2010) Psychosocial assessment and repetition of self-harm: The significance of single and multiple repeat episode analyses. *Journal of Affective Disorders*, 123, 95–101.

Beyers, J., Loeber, R., Wikstrom. P. and Stouthamer-Loeber, M. (2001) What predicts adolescent violence in better-off neighbourhoods? *Journal of Abnormal Child Psychology*, 29(5), 369–381.

Bhugra, D. and Desai, M. (2002) Attempted Suicide in South Asian Women. *Advances in Psychiatric Treatment*, 8, 418–423.

Biddle, L., Donovan, J., Owen-Smith, A., Potokar, J., Longson, D., Hawton, K. and Gunnell, D. (2010) Factors influencing the decision to use hanging as a method of suicide: Qualitative study. *British Journal of Psychiatry*, 197(4), 320–325.

Biskin, R. and Paris, J. (2012) The Diagnosis of Borderline Personality Disorder. *Canadian Medical Association Journal*, 184(16), 6 November, 1789–1794.

Brezo, J., Paris, J., Vitaro, F., Hebert, M., Tremblay, R.E. and Turecki, G. (2008) Predicting suicide attempts in young adults with histories of childhood abuse. *British Journal of Psychiatry*, 193, 134–139.

Buckland, L. (2011) Nearly a million Russians have committed suicide since collapse of Soviet Union. *Daily Mail*, 24 October.

Callaghan, P. and Waldcock, H. (eds.) (2006) *The Oxford Handbook of Mental Health Nursing*. OUP: Oxford.

Cao, L., Zhao, J. and Van Dine, S. (1997) Prison disciplinary tickets: A test of the deprivation and importation models. *Journal of Criminal Justice*, Elsevier, 25(2), 103–113.

Carter, G., Page, A., Large, M., Hetrick, S., Milner, J.A., Bendit, N., Walton, C., Draper, B., Hazell, P., Fortune, S., Burns, J., Patton, G., Lawrence, M., Dadd, L., Dudley, M., Robinson, J. and Christensen, H. (2016) Royal Australian and New Zealand College of Psychiatrists clinical practice guideline for the management of deliberate self-harm. *Australian and New Zealand Journal of Psychiatry*, 50, 939–1000.

Case, A. and Deaton, A. (2020) *Deaths of Despair and the Future of Capitalism*. Princeton, NJ: Princeton University Press.

Centre for Social Justice (2018) Desperate for a Fix. The Centre for Social Justice. www.centreforsocialjustice.org.uk.

Clark, D. (2022) Number of police recorded non-sexual crimes of violence in Scotland from 2002/03 to 2020/21. www.statista.com.

Clements, C., Turnbull, P., Hawton, K., Geulayov, G., Waters, K., Ness, J., Townsend, E., Khundakar, K. and Kapur, N. (2016) Rates of self-harm presenting to general hospitals: a comparison of data from the Multicentre Study of Self-Harm in England and Hospital Episode Statistics. *BMJ Open*, 16(2), February, e009749. DOI: 10.1136/bmjopen-2015–009749. PMID: 26883238; PMCID: PMC4762081.

Cooper, J., Kapur, N., Webb, R., Lawlor, M., Guthrie, E., Mackway-Jones, K. and Appleby, L. (2005) Suicide after deliberate self-harm: A 4-year cohort study. *American Journal of Psychiatry*, 162, 297–303.

Cutliffe, J. (2005) Assessing risk of suicide and self-harm. In: Barker, P. (ed.) *Psychiatric and Mental Health Nursing: The craft of caring*. London: Routledge.

Crown Prosecution Service (2022) Homicide: Murder and Manslaughter. www.cps.gov.org.

Daffern, M., Howells, K. and Ogloff, J.R.P. (2007) The interaction between individual characteristics and the function of aggression in forensic psychiatric inpatients. *Psychiatry, Psychology and Law*, 14, 17–25.

Dawson, J.M. and Langan, P.A. (1994) Murder in families. US Department of Justice, Office of Justice Programs, Bureau of Justice Statistics.

Das, S. (2019) How strong is the link between mental health and crime? *GQ*, 22 June.

De Vogel, V., de Ruiter, C., Bouman, Y. and de Vries, Robbe M. (2012) *SAFROV Guidelines for the Assessment of Protective Factors for Violence Risk*. Utrecht: Forum Educatief.

Dennis, M.S., Wakefield, P., Molloy, C., Andrews, H. and Friedman, T. (2007) A study of self-harm in older people: Mental disorder, social factors and motives. *Aging & Mental Health*, 11(5), 520–525. DOI: 10.1080/13607860601086611.

Deonna, A.J., Rodogno, R., and Teroni, T. (2011) *In Defence of Shame: The Faces of an Emotion*. New York: Oxford University Press.

Department of Health (2002) *National Suicide Prevention Strategy for England: annual report on progress*. London: DoH.

Dixon-Gordon, K., Harrison, N., and Roesch, R. (2012) Non-Suicidal Self-Injury Within Offender Populations: A Systematic Review, *International Journal of Forensic Mental Health*, 11(1), 33–50. DOI: 10.1080/14999013.2012.667513.

Ducharme, J. (2019) Suicide Deaths Are Often 'Contagious.' This May Help Explain Why. *Time Magazine*, 18 April.

Durcan, G. (2021) *The Future of Prison Mental Health Care*. London: Centre For Mental Health.

Evans, L. (2011) Murder Rate: the trends that solve the crime. *The Guardian*, 20 January.

Fanning, J.R., Berman, M.E., Mohn, R.S. and McCloskey, M.S. (2011) Perceived threat mediates the relationship between psychosis proneness and aggressive behavior. *Psychiatry Research*, 186(2–3), 30 April, 210–218. DOI: 10.1016/j.psychres.2010.09.010. Epub 20 October 2010. PMID: 20965573; PMCID: PMC3041859.

Farrington, D.P. and Nuttall, C.P. (1980) Prison Size, Overcrowding, Prison Violence, and Recidivism. *Journal of Criminal Justice*, 8, 221–231.

Faulkner, A. (1997) *Briefing No. 1 – Suicide and Deliberate Self-Harm*. Mental Health Foundation.

Gairin, I., House, A. and Owens, D. (2003). Attendance at the accident and emergency department in the year before suicide: Retrospective study. *The British Journal of Psychiatry*, 183(1), 28–33.

Gardner, K.J., Dodsworth, J., and Selby, E.A. (2014) Borderline personality traits, rumination, and self-injurious behavior: An empirical test of the emotional cascades model in adult male offenders. *Journal of Forensic Psychology Practice*, 14(5), 398–417.

Gawande, A. (2020) Why Americans Are Dying from Despair. *The New Yorker*, March.

Gelder, M., Mayou, R. and Cowen, P. (2001) *Shorter Oxford textbook of psychiatry*. Oxford: Oxford University Press.

Gil, N. (2017) True Number Of UK Suicides May Be Far Higher Than Reported. MIND, 6 January. See www.refinery29.com.

Gilligan, J. (1997) *Violence: Reflections on a National Epidemic*. New York: Vintage Books.

Giupponi, G. and Machin, S. (2022) Labour market inequality. *IFS Deaton Review of Inequalities*, www.ifs.org.uk/inequality/labour-market-inequality.

Guthmann, E. (2005) The Allure: Beauty and an easy route to death have long made the Golden Gate Bridge a magnet for suicides. *The San Francisco Chronicle*, October 30.

Guthrie, E., Kapur, N., Mackway-Jones, K., Chew-Graham, C., Moorey, J., Mendel, E., Marino-Francis, F., Sanderson, S., Turpin, C., Boddy, G., Tomenson, B. and Patton, G.C. (2001) Randomised controlled trial of brief psychological intervention after deliberate self poisoning. *British Medical Journal*, 323(7305), 135–137.

Harer, M.D. and Steffensmeier, D.J. (1996) Race and Prison Violence. Criminology, 34(3), August, 323–355.

Harris, C. and Barraclough, B. (1997) Suicide as an Outcome for Mental Disorders. *British Journal of Psychiatry*, 170, 205–228.

Harrison, A. and Hart, C. (eds.) (2006) *Mental Health Care for Nurses: Applying mental health skills in the general hospital*. Oxford: Blackwell.

Hart, C., Colley, R. and Harrison, A. (2009) *Risk Assessment Matrix: a screening tool for assessing risk in A&E Departments*. Kingston: Kingston University & St George's University of London.

Harty, M., and Walsh, J., (2018) Transforming Services for Forensic Patients. NHS England. https://www.england.nhs.uk/blog/transforming-services-for-forensic-patients/.

Hawton, K. (2005) Psychosocial Treatments Following Attempted Suicide. In: Hawton, K. (ed.) *Prevention and Treatment of Suicide: from science to practice*. Oxford: OUP.

Hawton, K. and James, A. (2005) Suicide and deliberate self-harm in young people. *British Medical Journal*, 330, 891–894.

Hawton, K., Casey, D., Bale, E., Ryall, J., Geulayov, G. and Brand, F. (2013) Self-Harm in Oxford. The University of Oxford, Centre for Suicide Research.

Health Foundation (2006) Statistics on Mental Health. www.mentalhealth.org.uk.

Henrikson, J.O. (2020) Violence, Shame, and Moral Agency – An Exploration of Krista K. Thomason's Position. *De Ethica. A Journal of Philosophical, Theological and Applied Ethics*, 6(1).

Her Majesty's Inspectorate of Probation (2021) *A joint thematic inspection of the criminal justice journey for individuals with mental health needs*. Manchester: Her Majesty's Inspectorate of Probation.

Hjelmeland, H., Hawton, K., Nordvik, H., Billi-Brahe, U., De Leo, D., Fekete, S., Grad, O., Haring, C., Kerkhof, J.F.M., Lonnqvist, J., Michel, K., Salandor Renberg, E., Schmidtke, A., Van Heeringen, K. and Wasserman, D. (2002) Why people engage in parasuicide: a cross-cultural study of intentions. *Suicide and Life-threatening Behavior*, 32, 380–393.

Hodgins, S. (2008) Violent behaviour among people with schizophrenia: a framework for investigations of causes, and effective treatment, and prevention. Royal Society Publishing.

Horne, O. and Csipke, E. (2009) From Feeling Too Little and Too Much, to Feeling More and Less? A Nonparadoxical Theory of the Functions of Self-Harm. *Qualitative Health Research*, 9(5).

Horrocks, J. and House, A. (2002) Self Poisoning and Self Injury in Adults, *Clinical Medicine*, 2, 509–512.

House of Commons Justice Committee (2021) Mental health in prison: Fifth Report of Session 2021–22. London: House of Commons.

House, A. and Owens, D. (2020) General hospital services in the UK for adults presenting after self-harm: little evidence of progress in the past 25 years. *Br J Psychiatry*, 217(6), December: 661–662. DOI: 10.1192/bjp.2020.85. PMID: 32368993.

Ireland, J.L. and Quinn, K. (2007) Officer attitudes towards adult male prisoners who self-harm: development of an attitudinal measure and investigation of sex differences. *Aggress Behav.*, 33(1), Jan–Feb, 63–72. DOI: 10.1002/ab.20168. PMID: 17441007.

Jeffrey, R. (1979) Normal Rubbish: deviant patients in casualty. *Sociology of Health and Illness*, 1(1), 90–107.

Karma, R. (2020) Deaths of Despair: the deadly epidemic that predated coronavirus. www.Vox.com.

King, M., Semlyen, J., See Tai, S., Killaspy, H., Osbourn, D., Popelyuk, D. and Nazareth, I. (2008) *Mental Disorders, Suicide and Deliberate Self-Harm in Lesbian, Gay and Bisexual People*. London: National Mental Health development Unit.

Kousoulis, A., Van Bortel, T., John, A., Morton, A. and Davidson, G. (2022) Coronavirus: Mental Health in the Pandemic Study. Mental Health Foundation. www.mentalhealth.org.uk.

Kulacaoglu, F. and Kose, S. (2018) Borderline Personality Disorder (BPD): In the Midst of Vulnerability, Chaos, and Awe. *Brain Sciences*, 8(11), November, 201.

Lader, D., Singleton, N. and Meltzer, H. (2000) *Psychiatric morbidity among young offenders in England and Wales*. London: Office for National Statistics.

Lanes, E. (2009) Identification of Risk Factors for Self-Injurious Behavior in Male Prisoners. *Journal of Forensic Sciences*, 54(3), 692–698. DOI: 10.1111/j.1556–4029.2009.01028.x.

Leib, K., Zanarini, M.C., Schmahl, C., Linehan, M. and Bohus, M. (2004) Borderline Personality Disorder. *Lancet*, 364, 453–461.

Linehan, M. (2009) Expert Answers on BPD. *The New York Times*, June 19.

Linehan, M. (2015) *DBT Skills Training Manual*. 2nd ed. New York, New York: Guilford Press.

Linehan, M. (2020) How Marsha Linehan Developed the Central Feature of Dialectical Behaviour Therapy. *Psychology Today*. www.psychologytoday.com.

Living Wage Foundation (2022) More than 3.5 people in low paid, insecure work. www.Living-wage.Org.uk.

Lohner, J. and Konrad, N. (2006) Deliberate self-harm and suicide attempt in custody: distinguishing features in male inmates' self-injurious behavior. *Int J Law Psychiatry*, 29(5), September–October, 370–385. DOI: 10.1016/j.ijlp.2006.03.004. Epub 19 June 2006. PMID: 16782200.

Lohner, J., and Konrad, N. (2007). Risk factors for self-injurious behaviour in custody: Problems of definition and prediction. *International Journal of Prisoner Health*, 3(2), 135–161. DOI: 10.1080/17449200701321654.

Maden, T. (2007) *Treating violence: a guide to risk management in mental health*. Oxford University Press: Oxford.

Main, T.F. (1957) The Ailment. *Psychology and Psychotherapy*, 30(3), The British Psychological Society, 129–145.

Markham, S. (2019) We have to learn from homicides committed by mental health patients. *BMJ Opinion*, 28 June.

Markham, S. (2020) Collaborative risk assessment in secure and forensic mental health settings in the UK. *General Psychiatry*, 33, e100291. DOI:10.1136/gpsych-2020–100291.

Marsh, I. (2014) Suicide: the hidden cost of the financial crisis. *New Statesman*, 5 August.

McCallion, H. and Farrimond, P. (2018) An independent review of the Independent Investigations for Mental Health Homicides in England (published and unpublished) from 2013 to the present day. www.england.nhs.uk.

McManus, M., Hassiotis, A., Jenkins, R., Dennis, M., Aznar, C. and Appleby, L. (2016) Suicidal thoughts, suicide attempts, and self-harm. In: McManus, S., Bebbington, P., Jenkins, R. and Brugha, T. (eds.) *Mental health and wellbeing in England: Adult Psychiatric Morbidity Survey 2014.* Leeds: NHS Digital.

McRae, I. and Westwater, H. (2022). What you need to know about UK inequality. *The Big Issue,* 21 June.

MIND (2021) Coronavirus: the consequences for mental health. www.MIND.org.uk.

Monahan, J., Steadman, H., Silver, E., Appelbaum, P., Robbins, P., Mulvey, E., Roth, L., Grisso, T. and Banks, S. (2001) *Rethinking risk assessment: The MacArthur study of mental disorder and violence.* New York: Oxford University Press.

Morgan, S. (2000) *Clinical Risk Management: a clinical tool and practitioner manual.* London: The Sainsbury Centre for Mental Health.

Mullen, P.E. (2000) Forensic Mental Health. *The British Journal of Psychiatry,* 176(4), April, 307–311. DOI: 10.1192/bjp.176.4.307.

Murphy, G.E. (1998) Why women are less likely than men to commit suicide. *Compr Psychiatry,* 39(4), July–August, 165–75. DOI: 10.1016/s0010–440x(98)90057-8. PMID: 9675500.

National Records of Scotland (2022) Drug related deaths in Scotland 2021. www.nrscotland. gov.uk.

National Institute for Clinical Excellence (2004) *Self-Harm: The short-term physical and psychological management and secondary prevention of self-harm in primary and secondary care.* Clinical Guideline 16, London: NICE.

NHS Centre for Reviews and Dissemination (1998) Deliberate Self-harm. *Effective Health Care,* 4(6), University of York: NHS Centre for Reviews and Dissemination.

NHS England (2021) Service Specifications: Adult Medium Secure Services including Access Assessment Service and Forensic Outreach and Liaison Services (FOLS). https://www.england. nhs.uk/wp-content/uploads/2018/03/Adult-Medium-Secure-Service-Specification-SCFT-WSBS-addendum-version.pdf.

NICE (2016) Physical Health of People in Prison. National Institute for Health and Care Excellence. https://www.nice.org.uk/guidance/ng57/chapter/recommendations.

Garnett, M.F., Curtin, S.C. and Stone, D.M., (2022) Suicide Mortality in the United States, 2000–2020. NCHS Data Brief, Number 433, March. Centre for Disease Control.

O'Brien, J. and Hart, C. (2013) *Clinical Risk Assessment and Risk Management.* London: South West London & St George's Mental Health NHS Trust.

O'Connor, R.C., Rasmussen, S. and Hawton, K. (2009) Predicting deliberate self-harm in adolescents: a six month prospective study. *Suicide and Life-Threatening Behavior,* 39, 364–375.

O'Connor, R.C. and Kirtley O.J. (2018) The integrated motivational-volitional model of suicidal behaviour. Phil. Trans. R. Soc. B 373: 20170268. DOI: 10.1098/rstb.2017.0268.

Office for National Statistics (2021) Deaths related to drug poisoning in England and Wales. www. ons.gov.uk.

Office for National Statistics (2022) Suicide by Occupation in England: 2011 to 2020. www.ons. gov.uk.

Office for National Statistics (2021) Mortality from leading causes of death by ethnic group, England and Wales: 2012 to 2019. www.ons.gov.uk.

Office for National Statistics (2022) Crime in England and Wales. www.ons.gov.uk.

Owens, D., Horrocks, J. and House, A. (2002) Fatal and Non Fatal Repetition of Self-harm: Systematic review. *British Journal of Psychiatry,* 181, 193–199.

Page, H. (2018) Team splitting and the 'borderline personality': a relational reframe. *Psychoanalytic Psychotherapy,* 32(3). www.tandfonline.com.

Paris, J. (2008) *Treatment of Borderline Personality Disorder: A Guide to Evidence-Based Practice.* The Guilford Press.

Pearson, A., Saini, P., Da Cruz, D., Miles, C., While, D., Swinson, N., Williams, A., Shaw, J., Appleby, L. and Kapur, N. (2009) Primary care contact prior to suicide in individuals with mental illness. *British Journal of General Practice*, 59, 825–832.

Pidd, H. (2014) Will Cornick: a model student who planned murder for three years. *The Guardian*, 3 November.

Phillips, M.R., Li, X. and Zhang, Y. (2002) Suicide rates in China, 1995–99. *The Lancet*, 359(9309), 9 March, 835–840.

Phillips, M.R., Yang, G., Zhang, Y., Wang, L., Ji, H. and Zhou, M. (2002a) Risk factors for suicide in China: a national case-control psychological autopsy study. *The Lancet*, 360(934730), November, 1728–1736.

Poulson, C. (2001) Shame: The Root of Violence. Presented at: The Standing Conference on Organizational Symbolism, Organization(s), Institutions and Violence. June 30th–July 4th, Dublin, Ireland.

Prison Reform Trust (2014) Prison Reform Trust Response to the Consultation on Preventing Suicide in England. London: Prison Reform Trust.

Putkonen, A., Kotilainen, I., Joyal, C.C. and Tiihonen, J. (2004) Comorbid personality disorders and substance use disorders of mentally ill homicide offenders: a structured clinical study on dual and triple diagnoses. *Schizophrenia Bulletin*, 30, 59–72.

Quinliven, L.M., Gorman, L., Littlewood, D., Monaghan, E., Barlow, S.J., Campbell, S.M., Webb, R.T. and Kapur, N. (2021) Relieved to be seen—patient and carer experiences of psychosocial assessment in the emergency department following self-harm: qualitative analysis of 102 free-text survey responses. *BMJ Open*, 11(5).

Ramchand, R., Gordon, J.A. and Pearson, J.L. (2021) Trends in Suicide Rates by Race and Ethnicity in the United States. *JAMA Network Open*, 4(5), e2111563. DOI: 10.1001/jamanetworkopen.2021.11563.

Ramluggun, P. (2013) A critical exploration of the management of self-harm in a male custodial setting: qualitative findings of a comparative analysis of prison staff views on self-harm. *J Forensic Nurs*, 9(1), Jan–March, 23–34. DOI: 10.1097/JFN.0b013e31827a5984. PMID: 24158098.

Recovery in the Bin (2016) A simple guide on how to avoid receiving a diagnosis of 'personality disorder'. *Clinical Psychology Forum*, 289, The British Psychological Society. https://explore.bps.org.uk/content/bpscpf/1/289/33.

Repper, J. and Perkins, R. (2003) *Social Inclusion and Recovery: a model for mental health practice*. London: Balliere Tindall.

Resnick, P.J. (2015) The Detection of Malingered Mental Illness. Presented at: U.S. Psychiatric and Mental Health Congress. September 10–13, San Diego.

Royal College of Psychiatrists (2006) *Self-harm*. London: RCP.

Royal College of Psychiatrists (2008) *Rethinking risk to others in mental health services. Final report of the scoping group*. London: RCP.

Savage, M. (2018) Loss of experienced staff leaving prisons unsafe. *The Guardian*, 29 April.

Scottish Government (2022) Homicide in Scotland 2020–21. www.gov.scot.

Seiden, R.H. (1978) Where are they now? A follow-up study of suicide attempters from the Golden Gate Bridge. *Suicide Life Threat Behaviour*, 8(4), Winter, 203–216. PMID: 217131.

Selby, E.A., & Joiner Jr, T.E. (2009) Cascades of emotion: The emergence of borderline personality disorder from emotional and behavioural dysregulation. *Review of General Psychology*, 13(3), 219–229.

Senior, M., Fazel, S. and Tsiachristas, A. (2020) The economic impact of violence perpetration in severe mental illness: a retrospective, prevalence-based analysis in England and Wales. *Lancet Public Health*, 5, e99–106.

Sentencing Council (2022) Disposals for offenders with mental disorders, developmental disorders or neurological impairments. www.sentencingcouncil.org.uk.

Shaw, C. and Proctor, G. (eds.) (2004) Women at the Margins: Special Issue on women and Border-line Personality Disorder. *Asylum magazine*, 4(3).

Siddique, H. (2014) Man reunited with stranger who talked him down from suicide attempt. *The Guardian*, 30 January.

Sinai, J., Schiller, T. and Wilmore, A. (2017) A KGH Pathway to Violence Model: Understanding Precursors to Becoming an Active Shooter. Keirnan Group Holdings. www.kiernan.co.uk.

Singleton, N., Meltzer, H., Gatward, R., Coid, J. and Deasy, D. (1998) *Psychiatric Morbidity Among Prisoners: Summary Report*. London: Office for National Statistics.

Slade, K., Edelmann, R., Worrall, M., and Bray, D. (2014). Applying the Cry of Pain Model as a predictor of deliberate self-harm in an early-stage adult male prison population. *LEGAL AND CRIMINOLOGICAL PSYCHOLOGY*, 19(1), 131–146. DOI: 10.1111/j.2044-8333.2012.02065.x.

Snow, L. (2002). Prisoners' motives for self-injury and attempted suicide. *The British Journal of Forensic Practice*, 4(4), 18–29.

Stene-Larsen, K. and Reneflot, A. Contact with primary and mental health care prior to suicide: A systematic review of the literature from 2000 to 2017. *Scand J Public Health*, 47(1), February, 9–7. DOI: 10.1177/1403494817746274. Epub 5 December 2017. PMID: 29207932.

Stompe, T., Ortwein-Swoboda, G. and Schanda, H. (2004) Schizophrenia, Delusional Symptoms, and Violence: The Threat/Control-Override Concept Reexamined. *Schizophrenia Bulletin*, 30(1).

Stueve, A. and Link, B.G. (1998) Gender differences in the relationship between mental illness and violence: Evidence from a community-based epidemiological study in Israel. *Social Psychiatry and Psychiatric Epidemiology*, 33, SS61–SS67.

Swanson, J. W., Estroff, S., Swartz, M., Borum, R., Lachiotte, W., Zimmer C. and Wagner, R. (1997) Violence and severe mental disorder in clinical and community populations: The effects of psychotic symptoms, comorbidity, and lack of treatment. *Psychiatry*, 60, 1–22.

Sykes, G.M. (1958) *The Society of Captives: A Study of a Maximum Security Prison*. Princeton: Princeton University Press.

The Economist International (2018) Suicide is Declining Almost Everywhere. *The Economist*, November 24.

The MONEE Project (1999) AFTER THE FALL *The human impact of ten years of transition*. The UNICEF Innocenti Research Centre. www.unicef-irc.org.

Thomas, K. and Gunnell, D. (2010) Suicide in England and Wales 1861–2007: a time-trends analysis. *International Journal of Epidemiology*, 39(6), December, 1464–1475. DOI: 10.1093/ije/dyq094.

Thomason, Krista K. (2015) Shame, Violence, and Morality. *Philosophy and Phenomenological Research*, 91(1), 1–24.

Thomson, F., Sherring, S. and Garnham, P. (2010) *A Guide to the Assessment and Management of Risk*. London: Oxleas NHS Foundation Trust.

Thorneycroft, G. (2020) People with severe mental illness as the perpetrators and victims of violence: time for a new public health approach. *The Lancet*, 5, February. DOI: 10.1016/S2468-2667(20)30002-5.

United Nations Office on Drugs and Crime (2019) Global Study on Homicide, 2019 edition. www.unodc.org.com.

Wall, T. (2022) Hundreds of mentally ill prisoners denied urgent treatment in England. *The Guardian*, 10 May.

Williams, J.M.G., Crane, C., Barnhofer, T. and Duggan, D. (2005) Psychology and suicidal behaviour: elaborating the entrapment model. In: Hawton, K. (ed.) *Prevention and Treatment of Suicidal Behaviour: from science to practice*. Oxford: Oxford University Press.

Williams, J.M.G. and Pollock, L.R. (2001) Psychological aspects of the suicidal process. In: K. van Heeringen (ed.) *Understanding suicidal behaviour: The suicidal process approach to research, treatment and prevention*. Chichester: Wiley.

Williams, K. (2015) *Needs and characteristics of young adults in custody: Results from the Surveying Prisoner Crime Reduction (SPCR) survey.* London: Ministry of Justice.

Wortley, R. (2003) Situational crime prevention and prison control. In: Smith, M.J. and Cornish, D.B. (eds.) *Theory for practice in situational crime prevention. Crime Preventions Studies*, Vol. 16. Money, New York: Criminal Justice Press.

Wyllie, C., Platt, S., Brownlie, J., Chandler, J., Connolly, S., Evans, R., Kennelly, B., Kirtley, O., Moore, G., O'Connor, R. and Scourfield, J. (2012) Men, Suicide and Society: why disadvantaged men die by suicide. *Samaritans.* www.media.samaritans.org.

Zahl, D. and Hawton, K. (2004) Repetition of deliberate self-harm and subsequent suicide risk: long-term follow-up study in 11,583 patients. *British Journal of Psychiatry*, 185, 70–75.

Part 2
General principles of risk assessment

Identifying potential risk factors, or picking out current clinical risk indicators, only provides the information about actual risk to then be assessed. That assessment is completed when the likelihood and consequences of the person acting have been worked through, a formulation developed and a risk management plan is in place.

Although there will be occasions when assessments need to be undertaken over an extended period, an understanding of risk – as opposed to a comprehensive mental health assessment – can be gained in a relatively brief period of time by staff who have received appropriate education and training, even if they do not work in a mental health setting.

For example, with adequate training, Emergency Department (ED) nurses can conduct a mental health triage, incorporating a risk assessment, within 5–15 minutes with sufficient competence to make an accurate referral to specialist mental health teams. Similarly, paramedics trained in the process and structure of risk assessment can conduct a risk assessment and develop a risk management plan, referring to the appropriate agency, even if that is simply to ensure the patient is taken to the nearest ED for further assessment and treatment.

Many General Practitioners and others in primary care have great experience in mental health and assessments, and work in the community with people trying to cope with significant risks before making referrals to specialist mental health services. Others may need to seek advice. But all GPs and experienced clinicians in primary care can triage and assess patients, predicated on them having received sufficient training from mental health experts, having a triage or assessment framework and access to expert advice and clinical supervision.

Different approaches to risk assessment

There is a variety of approaches to assessment. However, the evidence strongly suggests that the most effective is the use of structured professional judgement, or structured clinical assessment (see below). Other approaches are mentioned in passing only so readers can consider which they currently use and their rationale for doing so.

Structured professional judgement, or structured clinical assessment

This is not a specific assessment instrument but combines:

- the evidence base for risk factors;
- an individual, structured patient assessment;

DOI: 10.4324/9781003171614-3

- a formulation;
- a risk management plan (Bouch & Marshall, 2005).

Using this approach your decision is informed by aspects of an actuarial approach and background information. However, the application of clinical judgement is also required, demonstrating:

- the ability to weigh up the information gained through the assessment itself against any clinical risk factors identified;
- integrating this within any algorithms prescribed by your organisation;
- using this combination of tools and information to come to a reasoned decision that addresses the key issues in the patient's situation.

The unstructured clinical approach

This is based on the clinicians' judgement alone, consequent to their assessment and without reference to assessment tools or clinical risk indicators etc. It is thus dependent on the clinician's experience, highly subjective and, therefore, not recommended (Bouch & Marshall, 2005; Maden 2007).

The actuarial approach

This stems from compiling and analysing statistics in the world of insurance for the purposes of calculating risks and, therefore, premiums. Forensic psychiatry first adapted its methodology to try and predict dangerousness and risk. It involves:

- formal assessment methods such as the use of assessment tools, e.g. the HCR-20;
- the use of clinical algorithms or protocols.

The actuarial approach follows 'objective' procedures to classify risk, looking at probability and predictability. For example, clinical algorithms are 'an explicit description of appropriate steps to be taken in the care of a patient with a particular problem', which should account for a full clinical history, with subsequent recommendations for diagnosis and/or treatment based on the data obtained. Algorithms include 'branching logic' which allow recommendations to be 'individualised according to the patient's age, gender and specific clinical findings' (Komaroff, 1982).

Of course, assessing the likelihood of dangerous behaviour in the context of mental health problems is not the same as assessing chest pain or simply basing a prediction of future behaviour on what has gone before. It involves a degree of clinical analysis and this should be taken into account when considering the reliability of using an actuarial approach, which is of very limited value on its own (Bouch & Marshall, 2005).

We clearly cannot predict the future but knowing as much as possible about someone's history and current situation allows us more insight into potential outcomes.

Making use of the information gained from assessment

The wider the sources of your information, the more opportunity there is to deliberate on potential risks. However, the absence of information must not be a barrier to making decisions when they are urgently required. Clinicians also need to be confident they are not pursuing information that will either be irrelevant or over complicate the decision-making process. In determining what will be useful, key factors include:

- accessing documented information and records about the individual's own history, particularly in relation to previous risk behaviours. This is best done in their original form wherever possible, rather than through second hand reports, e.g. looking at a contemporary account of a hospital admission rather than a subsequent reference to it in a later summary;
- a comprehensive interview aimed at gaining information about the person – it is important to note the difference between a face-to-face assessment and the significant limitations placed upon the clinician conducting a telephone triage or assessment, or using an online medium such as Microsoft Teams;
- exploring the individual's current situation, mental state and behaviour in the context of clinical risk indicators (see Table 1.5, page 39);
- obtaining corroborating information from those who know the patient, e.g. family members, carers, their GP, other health and social care professionals, other agencies such as the police;
- the use of rating scales and, if sanctioned by the team or service, validated assessment tools.

There is always the possibility of tension between the available time and need to be thorough. In assessing risk, it is essential that the quality of the work is not compromised and that, as a team, every effort is made to ensure the clinician undertaking the assessment has sufficient time to do it properly.

Determining the risk will then occur in the context of:

- your judgements based on this information;
- knowledge of risk indicators and how they relate to your assessment;
- your reaction, based on your experience and sense of the person, often, incorrectly, referred to as 'intuition' or a 'gut feeling' but tapping into what Aristotle termed 'phronesis', the knowledge assimilated through the process of experience, in this case repeated clinical assessments – see also Gladwell (2005) for an interesting discussion on this issue.

Translating the assessment into a risk formulation

This is discussed in detail in Part 4. But, at this stage, it should be noted that any assessment has to be accompanied by a formulation, as it is the formulation that is the bridge between the assessment and risk management plan. This should aim to answer the following questions:

- How serious is the risk?
- Is the risk specific or general?
- How immediate is the risk?
- How volatile is the risk?
- What specific treatment, and which management plan, can best reduce the risk?

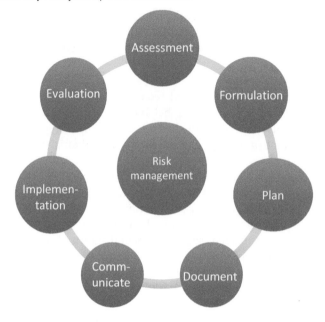

Figure 2.1 The formula for risk management

This requires having explored:

1. Who is at risk?
2. What is the risk?
3. How would they be at risk?
4. Where is the person(s) at risk?
5. When is the person(s) at risk?
6. Why is the person(s) at risk?

If these questions cannot be adequately answered, the assessment is incomplete.

Use the FACT principles in risk assessment

Fast
Accurate
Comprehensive
Therapeutic

The safety of the clinician and patient

In the community

Considering the risks that might affect the person needs to encompass the world in which they find themselves, rather than an idealised situation or one that would be suited to their needs. Some of these factors may be quite idiosyncratic to the individual so it's impossible to provide an exhaustive list. However, you should consider everything you think might be relevant.

Table 2.1 Safety and the referral process

Is the purpose of the referral clear?
Is it clear what the clinician/team are being asked to assess?
Have any known risks been clearly identified?
Is more information required?
Who should undertake the assessment – and why?
Ideally, where should the assessment take place?
How urgent is it?

For example, what potential risks are there in the wider environment? What, specifically, needs to be addressed? In any environment there will be a host of potential difficulties. For example, if substance misuse is a factor and there are drug dealers in the immediate neighbourhood, you need to consider how vulnerable the person is. If there are other particular risks in the person's locality, e.g. someone who might trigger dangerous behaviour to the patient and/or others, how will that be managed? Are there environmental factors that are more of a risk because of the person's impulsivity?

If prescribed medication is a crucial factor in the person remaining safe but they can't access a pharmacy without difficulty, that has to be factored into risk management. How will you ensure they have their medication? How will you know they're taking it?

Crucial to risk assessment is the safety of the clinician. Consideration of this begins from the moment information is being gathered through the referral process (see below). The referral should be reviewed by the clinical team wherever possible and a strategy devised to address any known or potential risks. If this is not undertaken by the team in a referrals meeting it should be delegated to a senior clinician who triages referrals on behalf of the team.

The next issue to consider is whether or not the environment is a safe one in which the assessment can take place. Issues discussed in other sections will also look at the impact of the assessment on the person and their safety, e.g. the clinician's ability to 'contain' the patient's anxiety and distress/disturbance, as well as the ability to minimise the patient's level of arousal. It's essential to monitor this throughout the interview and actively de-escalate the person if needed, even if this means not pursuing an element of the assessment as planned or even abandoning it altogether. Of course, this forms part of the assessment itself and contributes to a risk formulation and subsequent plan.

Because the risk is unknown when seeing a person newly referred, all first assessments outside of a clinical setting such as a health centre or hospital, e.g. someone's own home, should be undertaken by two people.

Key clinical tip

Under no circumstances should clinicians compromise their own safety. Take every opportunity to make the assessment process safe for yourself and it will be safer for the patient.

Before entering the person's home

Even before visiting the person's home, risk can be weighed:

- Is it safe for one person to visit on their own, remembering all initial assessments should be undertaken by two people?
- Is the surrounding area safe?
- If you are visiting by car, can it be parked to allow an easy and swift exit?
- What are the entrances/exit like? Can access and, particularly, egress be easily blocked?
- If the patient lives in a block of flats, what risks are there in the general environment?
- Do team members know exactly where you are, i.e. the patient's address?
- Have you informed the team of the time you are entering the premises and time you plan to finish?
- Check that you have adequate reception for your mobile phone before entering.
- By this time, before you enter, you will have effectively conducted a necessary 'doorstep assessment', which will determine whether or not you enter and conduct your full assessment.

Key clinical tip

If you have serious concerns about your safety do not enter the premises. If you begin to have concerns once you are in, provide a pre-rehearsed reason and leave immediately.

When entering the premises, do:

- Follow the person in rather than allowing them to remain by the door while you go in first. You don't want to find your exit blocked.
- Check the environment for potential weapons, while taking account of the likelihood they might be used. In someone's home, the kitchen is obviously a place where there are a lot of potentially dangerous things that could be used as weapons, e.g. knives. In other rooms, there will be any number of commonplace items that could be dangerous, but the key issue is how potentially dangerous you view the person you are assessing and whether or not there are any obvious weapons visible.
- Are there any others on the premises who might pose a potential risk? For example, you might know a particular family member has a history of violence. Equally, there may be people present you know nothing about, and weren't expecting to be there, while activity in the accommodation, such as drug taking, should be a prompt to leave immediately.
- Take a seat nearest the exit, wherever possible.
- Be mindful about discussing issues that lead to the patient becoming highly aroused beyond the point where you feel confident they can contain themselves or you can de-escalate the situation.
- Leave if the situation changes and you have serious doubts about your safety.
- Have a 'codeword' arranged with your team that can be used in an innocuous phrase, signalling you require immediate assistance. If you sense you are in potential danger and tell the patient you need to make a phone call telling someone you will be delayed,

this would allow you to use the word, e.g. it might be Osbourne, so saying, 'Please contact Mr Osbourne to let him know I'm running late…' will alert your colleagues that you need assistance.

- Have your mobile 'phone switched to speed dial for ready assistance.
- If you have concerns about the safety of the visit but have decided, on balance, to proceed with it, agree a time with the team by which you will have checked in with them, either in person or by phone, with a clear policy about what action is required and will happen if you don't.

Potential weapons

Almost any environment has a lot of potential weapons. Crucial questions are about which weapons the person has used before, has perhaps spoken about and their intent. Avoiding interviews where the person has immediate access to more obvious – and potentially lethal – weapons such as knives or very sharp implements is discussed in Part 2 (page 168).

However, it is worth remembering that immediate access to many things in anyone's house can be potentially dangerous. Some things are more obvious than others. A sharp weapon-like implement close to the person being interviewed can be picked up in the midst of a tense or heated discussion and hitting someone across the head can occur in a second, almost without thought.

If on a ward or inpatient unit/outpatient department

If the person is being admitted to a ward, how suited is that to the level of security required for that person, particularly if they may try to abscond? For someone at risk of suicide, are there obvious ligature points or areas of the ward where the person would be alone for long periods and risks potentially increased?

What is the dynamic like between patients on the ward? Is there anyone specific on the ward who might be either at risk from, or pose a danger to, the patient? Are there sufficient staff available, suitably skilled and experienced, to help the patient maintain their safety? Preparing for the assessment itself, consider:

- Who should carry out the assessment and how many staff should be involved in the actual assessment?
- If there is potential or known risk to others, have staff available for support if needed, having decided where they should be positioned, e.g. out of sight, outside the room, in the room etc.
- When doing an assessment on our own, ensure colleagues know:
  - any potential risks;
  - where you are;
  - what you're doing;
  - how long you will be – and what should happen if you encounter problems or are having problems exiting the room.
- Sit nearest the exit and within reach of alarm buttons.
- Place the chairs so they are a comfortable distance from one another and at an angle, which means you are not directly facing the patient but can easily establish eye contact (check to see if the patient is comfortable with the configuration).
- Minimise the potential for interruptions.

Systems, service structures and procedures

As outlined in Part 1, how our services are configured, access and availability will all be risk factors in themselves. Issues to consider include:

- If there is only a telephone triage system or helpline immediately available to the person, how will the assessor overcome the problems of not being able to see the person being assessed and compensate for the opportunity to assess body language, facial expression, congruity etc?
- If the crisis team will have to risk assess a known patient 'outside hours' or when that person is in crisis, what access do they have to the latest information about the person? How will they know they are acting consistently with previous risk management plans and can check out their proposals for a current risk management plan with the staff who will have to continue it?
- If there is pressure on beds or crisis services, how do clinicians arrive at rational decisions based on the assessment of the individual?

Communication and co-ordination

How issues around the assessment are communicated and co-ordinated is central to the risk management plan. A 'plan', no matter how good, cannot be considered to exist if it is not communicated to, and understood by, the appropriate people. If there are flaws or problems in communicating identified risk this will effectively nullify the impact of the assessment and potentially increase risk. As such, the clinician needs to know how effective communications systems are and factor these into the plan. For example:

- If clinicians responsible for managing the risk have a different record keeping system (often the case in Emergency Departments, prisons and areas where staff from different services work alongside each other), how will they know what you have written and planned? How will you ensure there is a record on their system as well as yours?
- If clinicians responsible for managing the risk won't have access to electronic records until the following day, what will you do to ensure the patient is safe until such time as they can read it and act upon it?
- If vital information has to be transmitted from one shift to another for several days, how will this be done?

  - Do clinicians have time to read the electronic records of all patients?
  - Do you have a system for identifying the people about whom there is the most concern?
  - Is this information displayed anywhere or is there a system for prioritising discussion to focus on them?
  - In an inpatient ward do you print off copies of safety care plans to ensure everyone can – and will – read them?

- If clinicians from a different team or service are to play an important role in the person's risk management, how will they know their specific responsibilities, what to do and what is in place in case things begin to go wrong?

If there are problems or, more specifically, gaps in any of these areas, this will adversely impact upon the risk management plan and effectively means it needs to be rewritten to take this into account.

In prison

Undertaking any type of assessment in prison is almost always difficult. Having access to a suitable room for a long enough period and the resident without custodial staff present is usually subject to the requirements of the prison regime or schedule. Wider considerations of security need to be balanced against the needs of the individual resident. Building a good relationship with custodial staff and working to ensure they understand the needs of the healthcare team in the prison is, therefore, an integral part of this process.

It's quite possible, if there is concern the resident is suicidal or has self-harmed, that the initial risk assessment will be undertaken as part of the Assessment, Care in Custody and Treatment (ACCT) procedure (a formalised risk assessment and risk management process unique to prisons, with standardised tools and documentation). As this is a prison process it will be led by a trained ACCT assessor – usually an officer from the prison – but they should be accompanied by a member of the healthcare team who should actively participate in the assessment. If the resident has had previous contact with healthcare, the team member should have an awareness of that contact, anything known about their history and, hopefully, be known to the resident.

As rooms and spaces suitable for interviews of this nature are usually in short supply, consider booking a venue, unless it is an emergency, and delaying the interview until it is available. Again, discuss with custodial staff all aspects of safety. Does an officer or officers need to be present? In the prison, the resident will have an 'unlock' status, i.e. a stipulated number of officers required to be present when the resident comes out of their cell. If there are officers required to be present it will inevitably complicate the assessment, potentially leaving the person more reluctant to talk about sensitive issues and worried about confidentiality.

These issues should be discussed openly and information given about the processes that govern the situation and the resident's concerns addressed.

There are occasions when risk assessments have to be conducted 'through, or at, the door', i.e. with the cell door shut and talking to the resident through the hatch. Again, risk to the clinician needs to be weighed up. Is it safe to have the hatch down and be talking to the resident? If not, because they pose a risk to others but also pose a risk to themselves, is there any way to balance these factors and explore the risk safely? If this isn't possible and there's sufficient concern, officers may need to remove all potentially dangerous items from the cell. Transfer to a safer environment might need to be considered, e.g. a safe cell that is free of ligature points or even an inpatient unit if there is one in the prison. Although this is a decision of senior custodial staff, healthcare staff should be prepared to make a recommendation based on whatever clinical information is available.

Taking a referral

The purpose of taking a referral is to gather as much information in advance of the assessment as possible.

Receiving 'good' or helpful referrals requires having a simple, easily understood process to enable clinicians – and patients, if self referrals are accepted – to access your service. If there are exclusion criteria these should be clear and have a sound rationale, along with information signposting the referrer to a service that can address their needs. For patients contacting the service directly it is even more important this is dealt with swiftly and effectively. The information a service requires in a referral should be clear but a lack of the desired information should not be an obstacle to seeing the person referred if it is clear there is significant risk involved. Engaging with the referrer in direct discussion to gain necessary further information not only enables the assessment to go ahead more quickly than if there is a lengthy but indirect back and forth about what is required, it also helps the referrer when making future referrals.

However, it is fundamental for effective services to have as few barriers as possible. For example, arbitrary definitions of 'crisis' or referral criteria that do not match service need may create delays, confusion and further problems and become a significant risk factor in themselves.

The referrer's perception of the urgency or immediacy of the referral has to be acknowledged and addressed, with appropriate levels of support and assistance offered to help them and the patient, whether or not the person will be seen as quickly as the referrer initially thinks necessary. Assisting the referrer in understanding available resources and what they can do to address the situation prior to the patient being seen is an important part of the process.

Issues that referrers should be made aware of as being helpful include:

- any known specifics about risk, current, in the past and potential. If there is unsubstantiated speculation about possible risk, this should also be considered;
- if a previous risk assessment has been carried out and is available to the referrer, you should expect to receive a copy in advance of seeing the patient. However, this should not be thought to exclude the need to do a new risk assessment or even a full assessment, remembering context and circumstances are different and the person's internal view of their past and personal history may have changed. Also, there may have been significant changes to their circumstances that have impacted upon risk and of which the referrer may have no knowledge;
- what, exactly, the referrer sees as the purpose of the referral and any action they expect to be taken, as well as any future involvement they would expect to have.

Use the STAR principles in taking a referral

The referral process should be:
Simple
Transparent
Accessible
Rapid

Gathering information

The patient should be regarded as the relevant expert in their life and the principle source of any information, which can be gained through a face-to-face interview. The importance of this is not just in conversation but direct observation, noting the congruence of what is said, tone of voice, body language and posture. When discussing attitudes and feelings, it has been estimated that only seven per cent is communicated through the content of *what* is said, with 38 per cent arising from *how* it is said, e.g. tone of voice, and the final 55 per cent through body language, e.g. facial expression, gestures, posture and body movement (Mehrabian, 1981).

Though the amount of communication through body language will vary when different themes are being communicated, the ability to see the person providing the information is obviously crucial when assessing serious risk. For example, there will be gestures and nonverbal acts that illustrate or emphasise particular points the person is talking about; affect displays or facial configurations will reveal emotional states that may be related or unrelated to the topic of discussion and are often unconscious. Gestures associated with this are often spontaneous and can be a better guide to how the person is feeling than what they are saying (Hannagan, 2007).

Working with families/carers and issues of confidentiality

Listening to the views of carers, relatives and friends who know the person well is crucial. The same is true within healthcare teams. The staff with most knowledge of the patient may be the healthcare assistant or support worker who spends the most time with them. This might include:

- information about their own relationship with the patient;
- the person's relationship with fellow patients and relatives when they visit;
- how they spend their time during the course of the day and if there is any change to their clinical presentation during the course of 24 hours;
- how they react to interactions with other colleagues, e.g. pre and post ward rounds;
- how they react to medication.
- Are there any issues, events or people who make things better or worse for the patient?

Carers can also be an invaluable support and be an integral part of a risk management plan. However, several factors need to be considered, including:

- carers should not be overburdened and given responsibilities which they are either not ready for or able to carry out;
- the patient may not wish to receive their support at this time;
- the carer may be at risk.

Supporting the patient and carers can often be a difficult balancing act but it is an integral part of the assessment and assumptions should not be made.

Further information and corroboration should be gained from patient records, family members, carers, health, social care or other professionals who have had contact with the patient.

Permission from the patient should be sought before seeking information from other sources but if there are serious concerns about the safety of the individual or others these outweigh issues of confidentiality and every effort should be made to obtain the information even if the individual hasn't agreed. Communicating serious concerns with other healthcare professionals and/or agencies about the safety of an individual and/or the public always supersede requirements about confidentiality.

Working constructively with carers and families is an essential part of the risk assessment and risk management process.[i] If families or friends are concerned that someone may be at risk it is important that they are able to voice their concerns and that these will be fully and objectively considered during the assessment process. As already noted, it has been widely recognised in many serious incident inquiries, including those after suicides and homicides, that carer and family concerns were not given sufficient credibility nor warnings from them heeded by clinical teams.

Equally, they should be given information and support as soon as possible. Even when it is clear there are significant risk issues, family or friends may fear saying the wrong thing. It is useful for you to establish as early as possible what information, if any, the patient is willing to share with relatives and/or carers (O'Brien and Hart, 2013). However, supporting families by providing general advice does not break confidentiality, as is shown in the examples below:

Example 1: *"I can't speak to you about your daughter without her permission, but I can tell you if someone has a condition such as you've described, these are the symptoms to look out for..."*

Example 2: *"If you're worried about your daughter experiencing this, or maybe beginning to experience this, then please call the team on this number..."*

Key clinical tip

In many suicide and homicide inquiries, it has emerged that the concerns of family members and/or carers were not given sufficient importance. Their input should be a key consideration in your assessment.

Note

i   Family members are often the main carers. If carers and/or family members have a role in any risk management plan, it is important that they have agreed to this and their role is clear to everyone, including the patient. It's also essential the clinical team are confident family members/carers are able to undertake the role allocated to them. This should be documented in the risk management plan and all relevant parties should have a copy of this plan. Family members may be at increased risk in some instances from the patient and this needs to be incorporated into any risk management strategy.

References

Bouch, J. and Marshall, J.J. (2005) Suicide risk: structured professional judgement. *Advances in Psychiatric Treatment*, 11, 84–91.

Department of Health (2011) *Consultation on Preventing Suicide in England: a cross-government outcomes strategy to save lives*. London: DoH.

Komaroff, A.L. (1982) Algoriths and the 'Art' of Medicine. *American Journal of Public Health*, 72(1), 10–12.

Gladwell, M. (2005) *Blink: The power of thinking without thinking*. London: Penguin.

Hannagan, T. (2007) *Management* (5th edition). London: Prentice Hall.

Harrison, A. (2006) Self-harm and suicide prevention. In: Harrison, A. and Hart, C. (eds.), *Mental Health Care for Nurses: Applying mental health skills in the general hospital*. Oxford: Blackwell.

Hawton, K., Harriss, L. and Zahl, D. (2006) Deaths from all causes in a long term follow up study of 11,583 deliberate self harm patients. *Psychological Medicine*, 36, 397–405.

Maden, T. (2007) *Treating violence: a guide to risk management in mental health*. Oxford University Press: Oxford.

Mehrabian, A. (1981). *Silent messages: Implicit communication of emotions and attitudes* (2nd edition). Belmont, California: Wadsworth.

Morgan, S. and Wetherell, A. (2009) Assessing and managing risk. In: Norman, I. and Ryrie, I. (eds.), *The Art and Science of Mental Health Nursing* (2nd edition). Berkshire: OUP.

O'Brien, J. and Hart, C. (2013) *Clinical Risk Assessment and Risk Management*. London: South West London & St George's Mental Health NHS Trust.

Part 3
Undertaking a risk assessment

Potential barriers

Before beginning an assessment, consider any potential barriers to communication that might affect the process and what steps can be taken to mitigate these. They may include:

- someone having a learning disability;
- disruption to the person's perception;
- language;
- literacy;
- culture and health beliefs;
- culture and gender beliefs;
- culture and lack of understanding.

If any of these factors have been identified in advance, seek ways to address them, e.g. getting specialist advice about assessing someone with the specific learning disability your patient has, the use of an interpreter, considering how you will provide materials for someone with a literacy problem or work with an individual's cultural difference.

Considering language focuses on more than dialect or the spoken communication of a particular nation. You also need to think about the person's ability to articulate their inner world, their thoughts and, particularly, feelings.

The person may come from a community where there is distrust of mental health services. As an individual they may have particular beliefs about health, e.g. homeopathic medicine is best, psychiatric medication is harmful. There may be cognitive 'rules' to which they subscribe, e.g. 'We don't talk about our feelings'; 'You should be able to sort out your own problems' etc.

These will have to be addressed within the assessment but also should feature as a part of the assessment itself and figure in your formulation and plan.

First impressions

Having established a safe environment and provided the person being assessed with sufficient information about the process, the formal part of the assessment starts. An important issue arises from your very first impression on seeing the person. This may be

DOI: 10.4324/9781003171614-4

as you walk into the reception area of a health centre, a room on a ward or into the person's house.

Texts about risk assessment focus on careful, nuanced, in-depth analysis and decision making. Yet, first impressions often create an instant response and, whether or not we welcome them, can have a powerful impact on our judgement (Gladwell, 2005). Are these trustworthy? Research undertaken into the adaptive unconscious strongly suggests first impressions can tell us a lot about someone and/or a situation (and there is even richer 'information' when the first meeting is in the person's home).

The kind of observations that might be useful include:

- What is the person's facial expression and demeanour?
- What, specifically, did you notice?
- What were they doing at the moment you saw them?
- Did they make eye contact or look away?
- Did they change their posture and, if so, in what way?
- Did their breathing change?
- Did they immediately start talking?
- Did the person meet your expectations – and what were those expectations?
- How did you feel, and what was it about the person that led you to feel that way? For example, if you suddenly felt anxious, what caused that?
- Most importantly, was that first impression borne out by what you learned about the person during the rest of the assessment?
- If not, what was different?

As useful as this might be, however, this initial impression might tap into unconscious negative attitudes or even prejudices, e.g. about 'people who self-harm', and might influence the interaction without the clinician being aware. The clinician may also 'follow' their first impression about the patient, seeking information that reinforces it and not looking to establish as broad a picture as might otherwise have been the case. Cultural differences might account for the person not meeting preconceptions.

Clinicians always need to be aware of the limitations of their knowledge of other cultures and potential unconscious bias before carefully balancing their first impression with an in-depth assessment. Practice – the act of undertaking risk assessments, building from being supervised to either doing them alone or leading in the process but doing so frequently and regularly – assists in the development of what Aristotle termed phronesis, usually translated as practical wisdom or prudence. Aristotle noted that certain types of knowledge can only become known through experience rather than teaching or formal learning. It has also been termed innominate knowledge. This has been described as knowledge that is derived from practice, experience, doing things over and over, rather than theory or organised study. It is what is often – wrongly – termed 'intuition'. This is the type of rapid decision making that experienced people in many different walks of life exercise, apparently 'on a hunch' or a 'gut feeling' but which is actually more likely the result of having gone through the same process so many times that every nuance and the many small signs that might not be recognisable by a less experienced practitioner are noticed, where the incongruence of someone's body language or facial expression with their verbal response immediately rings alarm bells or satisfies the clinician that what they are hearing is likely to be an accurate reflection of how the person is actually feeling and thinking.

Key clinical tip

Make a careful mental note of your first impression, while being mindful of any potential prejudices.

Initial communications and developing a rapport

It is never safe to assume you have a willing partner in the assessment. Gauging the patient's degree of collaboration is integral in determining the risk. However, this is not a static process. The way in which the clinician builds and develops a rapport and seeks the individual's collaboration and agreement in the assessment process is crucial to how the risks change. Feeling comfortable and engaged in the process is likely to help the person talk more freely about their experiences and seek helpful solutions while interpersonal problems experienced in the early stages of an interview will undoubtedly complicate the process and make it more difficult. Picking up on the person's cues is an essential part of this (see below).

Helping the person understand the purpose of the interview and how it will be conducted will assist in developing a rapport (see Table 3.1). A collaborative process also involves the clinician 'entering the world' of the patient, however 'disturbed' this might be, embracing the person's current experience and exploring it without judgement or prejudice. An empathic acceptance of the patient's experience and communicating that their responses can be understood and make sense within the context of their background and/or current circumstances can be invaluable (Linehan 1993).

How does this work in practice? One example might be in talking with someone about their beliefs about a conspiracy to harm them. It may be difficult to understand as they describe plots to harm them and unseen forces at work to do things they believe place them in serious danger. However, without colluding with delusional beliefs or anything dangerous or potentially illegal, it both validates the person's experience and provides invaluable information for the clinician to be curious about this world, to want to understand how it works, how the person makes sense of what is happening and how they *feel* as a consequence, as well as what they have decided to do because of what is 'happening'.

If the person is compliant simply because they fear a more coercive response from the clinician should they be obviously resistant, e.g. detention under the Mental Health Act, this is *not* concordance and interventions should be gauged accordingly (see Figure 3.1).

Table 3.1 Information to provide to the patient at the start of the assessment

The purpose and nature of the interview
Approximately how long it will take/how much time you have available
Explain that you will be asking a number of questions, more than will be the case in any future sessions - if you expect to be seeing the person again - and that some may be potentially 'difficult' questions, also giving the rationale for this
Questions don't have to be answered but it is helpful to do so
There will be an opportunity for the patient to ask questions
What will happen with the information provided
What happens next and when

Identifying reasons for non-compliance, if present, are as important as anything else in the assessment and makes any response and attempt to improve collaboration more effective. Reasons could include:

- lack of 'insight' or disagreeing with the wider understanding and interpretation of the person's mental state, behaviour or view of the world;
- the person may have incorporated you and/or the assessment into a wider paranoid belief system;
- denial or minimisation of the problem;
- guilt;
- something they reveal may have unwanted consequences for them;
- shame;
- a desire to maintain control and independence;
- instrumental reasons, i.e. they want something from the interview they don't think they can achieve by collaborating fully with you.

While it is important to seek permission as part of the collaborative process and offer the individual the option of not answering questions that cause distress or are uncomfortable, you need to think through how to try and access information the person is unwilling or finding it difficult to impart. For example:

- Have you asked too probing a question too early?
- Does the person understand what you mean?
- Could you have phrased the question better?
- Does the person feel too embarrassed to answer?
- Is it too distressing to answer?
- Is the person being evasive?
- Are they unwilling to co-operate with you?

There is a possibility that, if you are unable to obtain the information to enable you to make a reasoned judgement and decision with the person about managing the risk, you will need to consider more restrictive options.

How might the degree of collaboration be assessed in the risk assessment?

- How did the person come to be interviewed, e.g. were they detained by the police or brought unwillingly? Did they seek help themselves?
- Do they offer information in the interview itself or are their answers monosyllabic and/or evasive?
- Does what they say corroborate other information you have?
- Is the content of what they tell you consistent throughout or does it change in response to different questions?
- Is the content of their account of their mental state consistent with what you would expect, from what you know of any diagnosed or probable mental health problems?
- Is there congruence between what is said, body language and behaviour?
- Are they engaged throughout?
- Are they willing to see you again if necessary or in agreement with a plan that you think will help them and/or others stay safe? Can they give a plausible account of how they will meet the conditions of that plan?

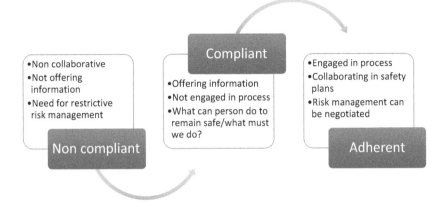

Figure 3.1 The relationship between the degree of collaboration and the risk management plan

---

Key clinical tip

Good communications skills help develop a rapport. Using this rapport from the outset allows you to help the person tell their story and can promote thinking about solutions even while taking an apparently problem dominated history.

Establishing psychological safety and developing a rapport – skills needed

Creating psychological safety within the interview will help the person feel able to ask for help, find it easier to open up about difficult issues, raise concerns, listen to comments and observations from the interviewer and challenge their own thinking and behaviour.

This involves trying to exchange neutral information in the opening stages of the interview process and avoiding the person feeling exposed, encouraging them to talk to you about something which is 'safe' and not challenging in any way. Aim to ask 'safe' questions not related to the assessment, taking cues from the environment or situation so the person is used to responding to you (see clinical example 1).

However, this is the beginning of developing a 'therapeutic relationship', something quite specific and unique to healthcare. Whether sitting down in a clinical situation with an individual you haven't met before or meeting someone who is well known to you through your clinical practice, this should always be your ultimate aim.

As noted by Reynolds (2003), 'the therapeutic relationship is not a nebulous, kind hearted, well intentioned relationship'. For the purposes of this *Pocket Guide*, there is no need to go into this in great detail but it is worth thinking about how this enables the risk assessment to proceed as easily as possible. Stuart (2005) defines it as, 'a mutual learning experience and a corrective emotional experience for the patient'. The clinician will use 'personal attributes and clinical techniques in working with the patient' to 'enable them to learn more satisfactory and productive patterns of behaviour' (Reynolds, 2003).

An early stage of building any new relationship, often termed the orientation phase, is to develop a *rapport*. It is important to distinguish between the skills required for building a rapport with someone you don't know, for what is likely to be a 'one off' contact, from those used to develop a therapeutic relationship over the longer term, as there are subtle differences to the skills and process.

Building a rapport involves skills familiar to most healthcare staff. It begins with shifting from the neutral topics to establish psychological safety to seek common ground – the most important aspect of this is the way in which the clinician focuses on the person being assessed, using the techniques outlined below. It can also mean picking up on 'small things', such as shared interests, commenting on aspects of the person's experience and story that are not necessarily clinically relevant.

'Active listening" is defined in different ways but involves concentrating on what is being said, comparing it with the nonverbal messages coming from the person and absorbing and processing it. Doing this not only helps you better understand them and creates a mutuality between you and the person you're listening to, it makes it possible to pick up on important cues in what they're telling you. This is in itself a demonstration that you're actively listening, but also encourages further cues and greater openness from the person. If these initial cues are missed, it is likely the person will offer fewer and fewer as the interview continues.

One thing that should almost always be shared is the desire to find a solution to the current 'problem,' 'need' or reason the person is with you at that moment, as well as then helping that person 'move on'. Of course, there may well be disagreement about how, and how quickly, that will happen. Nonetheless, to make this a stated purpose of the assessment can often be helpful (and it may not be clear to the person being assessed unless explicitly said), after which the clinician's negotiating skills may well be required to give it genuine meaning for the person.

An approach that will enable the building of a rapport will include demonstrating:

- courtesy and respect for the person, even if the person is quite challenging or uncooperative;
- interest in the person's story;
- empathy;
- building trust by being:

  - honest;
  - clear about the purpose of the contact;
  - genuine – using your own language, avoiding jargon, being as open as possible;
  - giving information.

However, it also involves some skills that we might use, but not necessarily knowingly.

Pacing

This is a means of connecting with the other person and communicating a sense of understanding. It means 'entering' the other person's world by:

- listening to and observing the other person carefully;
- reflecting what he or she knows and regards as important and true and matching some part of their ongoing experience

For example, replying to someone who doesn't want to take medication because of its side effects, you might say, "A lot of people share that view and some medications are known to have very unpleasant side effects." This is not you agreeing with them but seeking common ground.

We can pace a person's mood, body language and speech patterns, including tone, volume and the type of words, phrases and images that person uses. You can even pace their breathing patterns as a way of building a rapport. You obviously do not want to be as loud or physically active as someone who is very aroused and behaving in a disturbed or distressed manner; nor would you want to be as slowed down and psychologically retarded as a depressed person. However, pacing as much as possible allows you to gradually exert influence over the other person, either by slowing down the communication with the aroused person or subtly lifting the depressed person, bringing them closer to your pace.

Mirroring

This is about reflecting back to the person something we see and understand about them. It involves getting into rhythm with the person on as many levels as possible, e.g. adopting something of the way they talk, sitting the way that they sit, using the same gestures and body language, moving in the general pattern that they are moving, having a similar expression. All of these things communicate a sense of understanding the person, of connection, making it more likely they will share more information.

As the conversation progresses, if these techniques are working and you are connecting on an emotional level, you would expect the person to start mirroring you. Both pacing and mirroring can allow you to start leading as the conversation progresses. If you are not seeing any mirroring from the other person then it is unlikely that connection is deepening and you may need to rethink how you are communicating, although it may also indicate something about the person's current mental state or personality.

Clinical Example 1:   Giving information and developing a rapport

Clinician: Hello, William, as I said at the door and we put in our letter, my name is John and this is my colleague, Sarah. We're from the Community Mental Health Team, based at the local mental health centre. We see everyone referred to us from this area. Thanks very much for letting us come and visit you.

William: Yeah, well, I'm still not sure what you're here for.

Clinician: As I wrote in my letter, we've been asked by your GP–

William: [*Interrupts*] I saw that. But why does she want you to see me? What's it all for?

William: She asked us to see you because, as I understand it, you'd told her you were having trouble sleeping and have been having panic attacks. And some other experiences that you'd found worrying? Is that right?

William: Yeah, but I told her I'd be okay.

Clinician: It sounds as if you're reluctant to see us?

William: Absolutely. I didn't want to see you. And I told her that.

Clinician: That's not unusual, William. A lot of people are reluctant to see us. But those worries about not sleeping and the panic attacks were serious enough at the time for you to seek help?

William:	[*Pause*] Yes... and that's why I wanted some sleeping tablets, because I'm up all night and that was driving me nuts, same as the funny turns.
Clinician:	Are you still up all night and having funny turns?
William:	Yes. But I don't... I don't want to have to see anyone about it.
Clinician:	What particularly is worrying you about seeing us today?
William:	I don't want to end up back in hospital. And I've got the dog now. I couldn't leave her.
Clinician:	I've got a dog, They're great company, aren't they?
William:	[*Nods*]
Clinician:	But I guess they're a worry as well. Mine looks a little like yours but is a bit smaller. Yours has a lovely temperament. What's her name?
William:	Madonna. [*Smiles*]
Clinician:	Madonna? You a fan?
William:	Yes. But Kelly mainly.
Clinician:	Did you grow up with dogs in the family?
William:	Yeah. When I was a kid...
Clinician:	Where was that?
William:	Eh? South London. Tooting.
Clinician:	There's a market there, isn't there?
William:	There's three.
Clinician:	Was there a stall there that sold live eels?
William:	[*Chuckles*] Yeah. They used to frighten me when I was a kid. You been there?
Clinician:	Yeah. When I was a lot younger. But, back to you... You're worried if you talk to us, you might end up in hospital?
William:	I did last time.
Clinician:	Obviously neither Sarah or I knew you then, but I've had a chance to read your notes and I did see you were unhappy about being in hospital, so I'm not that surprised you're reluctant to talk to us today. But Dr Jones told me she didn't think she had the particular skills to really help you just now. She said she was very worried things were getting on top of you.
William:	She said that?
Clinician:	Yes. Which is why she got in touch with us. I'm happy to go at your pace. I thought we might look at ways in which we could help you prevent things getting any worse, like helping you get some sleep, and doing something about those funny turns, as well as talking about what's been happening recently.
William:	I'm not sure I'm ready for that.
Clinician:	Well, as I said, we can go at your pace. And it can't be a nice feeling to think you're going nuts in the middle of the night.
William:	It isn't.
Clinician:	Okay. I'll just tell you how we go about these conversations. It does involve a lot of questions as Sarah and I try to get to know something about you – though not all our meetings will be like this if we do agree to carry on meeting...

Key clinical tip

You have to work to develop a rapport, using a range of skills. Be attentive, actively listen and look for cues. Be aware of pacing and mirroring and ready to enter the person's 'world' to try and understand their perspective without colluding or saying things you don't believe to be true.

Nonverbal communication

So much that's written about assessment focuses on what is said yet, as we have noted, most of our communication is nonverbal. As we need to focus attention on the nonverbal communication of the patient, we also have to be aware not only of what we communicate without speaking but also how our body language, posture and physical presence can be used to assist the assessment process.

We should remember that most people being interviewed are likely to be experiencing some degree of anxiety, if not directly as a consequence of their mental state then in relation to being 'assessed,' which they may equate with being 'judged', or having possible negative outcomes.

It can, therefore, be 'containing', psychologically, for the person being interviewed if you are able to present yourself in a calm, thoughtful and open manner, be able to listen without judgemental comments or responses and set boundaries where required while being flexible enough to respond to the individual's needs (see section 3.2 below).

Always consider whether or not your **body language**, **facial expression** and **tone of voice** are congruent with what you are saying. If they're not, you need to consider why that might be the case:

- How are you feeling towards the patient?
- Is there something going on in the interview that you are finding difficult or feel uncomfortable about?
- Might it be something you 'brought in' with you from a previous session or outside work?
- How are you going to deal with it in the assessment, while you're with the patient?

Table 3.2 Putting the person at ease with your nonverbal communication and physical presence

Seating	Place the chairs you will use comfortably (when possible), angled at approximately 90°, so both people can make eye contact but not be looking directly at one another. Barriers, such as a table, should be removed if possible. It is also useful to simply ask the patient if they are comfortable with the seating arrangement – though you should always remember to place yourself in the chair with the easiest access to the exit and alarm buttons. In someone's home that may be difficult but should still be your aim.
Maintain eye contact	Even if the patient does not meet your gaze, continue to look at them. It both aids your own assessment of the person and, when they look back at you, will indicate your continued interest if your gaze is still there to be met.

Table 3.2 (Continued)

Build confidence and a sense of safety	Physically communicate your own *confidence* and sense of *safety* by appearing calm, by thinking about the situation and remaining engaged in the person's story, no matter how distressing.
Be patient	Allow the patient time to answer your questions. Don't rush. Even if you have another commitment, remain focused.

Key interview skills

There are a wide range of techniques that are going to be used in specific parts of an assessment. However, key aspects that will be used throughout, which are often a mix of verbal and nonverbal skills, will be useful in helping the person express difficult feelings and address difficult issues with you (see Box 8 below).

Box 8:   Key interview skills

- Have an interview structure with which you are familiar. It allows you to follow the person's story and facilitate digression if necessary but return to the important issues you need to explore.
- Employ active listening – communicate to the patient that you are both listening and interested in their story.
- Demonstrate empathy.
- Look for nonverbal cues:

  - Is there congruence between body language, facial expression and dialogue?
  - Does the person want you to pursue a line of inquiry?
  - Are they reluctant to answer a particular question?
  - Are they angry, sad, distressed?
  - Do they understand what you're saying?
  - If there is silence is it because they're not willing to respond, reflecting on what's been said already or thinking of what to say?

- Provide 'containment'.

Demonstrating empathy and compassion

Empathy is a complex, multi-dimensional response and cannot be 'acted'. It involves cognition, emotions and behaviour but also requires a focus on the other person through the careful use of observation.

Active or reflective listening leads to a cognitive process of reasoning and understanding, which in turn then has to be conveyed to the person to whom you are listening. This can be done in a variety of ways:

- Seeking to explore and clarify feelings, e.g. "How did you feel about your father's death?"

- Responding to feelings, e.g. "I'm sorry to hear that. It sounds as if it was very upsetting for you."
- Exploring the personal meaning of feelings, e.g. "You mentioned earlier that your dad died. What, exactly did you feel about that?"

Given that many people find it difficult to articulate their emotions, the ability to 'read' nonverbal cues such as body language, gestures, facial expression and tone of voice are key to intuiting others' emotions. It should come as no surprise then that nodding, the use of facial expression, pacing and mirroring will also demonstrate empathy. There is also evidence from exercises in studying the ability to 'read' others' expressions and nonverbal cues that has demonstrated that these are skills that can be learned through experience and exposure (Goleman, 1996). However, while you may see a physical response in the person that seems particularly important, don't make assumptions. It's better to point out what you've seen and ask about it, e.g. "I noticed that you became quite restless when you were talking about your dad. Was there a reason for that?"

Compassion, often quoted in nursing texts and cited in the Department of Health's Strategy and Vision for Nursing, Midwifery and Care Staff (Department of Health, 2012), is somewhat different to empathy. It is to recognise suffering in others and then take action to help them alleviate it. The active component of compassion – taking action – is the defining difference. It has religious connotations and the word derives from the Latin, meaning 'to suffer together'. It takes the clinician to a new, more active, phase in the relationship and is marked by the shift from risk assessment to risk formulation and risk management. This requires emotional labour (Smith, 1992), as well as emotional intelligence to use compassion-based interventions. It is for these reasons that reflective practice and clinical supervision are essential supports. There is evidence to suggest compassion-focused therapy can be particularly helpful for people experiencing shame and who are high in self-criticism (Leaviss and Uttley, 2015) and, while compassion in risk management is not a therapy in itself, its therapeutic value can be found in adopting a similar approach.

Containing the person's anxiety during the assessment

Containment is a very difficult concept to both grasp and practice but is simply defined by Casement (1985) as responding to 'times when people can't cope with their own feelings without assistance" and that the assistance being sought is "for *a person* to be available to help with these difficult feelings" (emphasis in the original). Casement also likens this process to:

- 'holding' the person in a psychological rather than physical sense;
- being available;
- offering understanding and, where appropriate, insight;
- being able to facilitate the person to talk about and then tolerate the feelings they find most difficult.

Clinical Example 2:   Containing the person's anxiety

Clinician: I notice when the subject of your dad's death came up you looked away, and you started rubbing your hands together. It's as if your

	whole body tightened up. Can you say what that's about?
William:	I can't talk about it.
Clinician:	Can you tell me what makes it so difficult?
William:	It's... the whole thing was just too awful.
Clinician:	I get the sense you think about this thing a lot, whatever it is, like it's going round and round in your head. So I'm not sure what would be different in talking about it. Do you worry what might happen if you say your thoughts out loud?
William:	Why would anyone want to hear about my problems?
Clinician:	Is that part of the reason you took the tablets?
William:	[*Long silence*] Yes. In part.
Clinician:	It sounds really...difficult, having thoughts that are so distressing but not feeling able to talk about them. Is there anything that might make it easier?
William:	What, to talk about how I couldn't wait for Dad to die, that all the time he was suffering I didn't really care, I just wanted it over?
Clinician:	Is it true you didn't care?
William:	It was just too much.
Clinician:	So, was it that you simply wanted him to die, or that you felt over-whelmed to see him suffer so much?
William:	I hadn't thought of it like that. It was... I don't know. Seeing him like that, it was just unbearable. I didn't know what to do to help him. I felt so helpless, like I was letting him down.

In this example, the clinician acknowledges and validates William's difficulty in articulating his feelings and possible fear it will be too much for the clinician to bear but continues to gently probe, aimed at helping him talk about what is troubling him.

The importance of containing the person's difficult feelings cannot be over emphasised. If they become physiologically aroused, the cognitive impact is that they will find it harder to think and participate fully. Moreover, this may lead them to cognitively interpret that arousal in ways that increase the likelihood of dangerous behaviours.

Therefore, as you probe deeper, you always need to be thinking of both how you can help the person express difficult feelings by the way you respond, while remaining composed and not becoming psychologically and physiologically overwhelmed yourself.

On another level, 'containment' is provided in those moments with a patient when, due to what is happening between you, you're experiencing powerful feelings – perhaps sadness, anxiety, even anger – but appear outwardly calm, in control and are able to process your emotions and not respond to them in unhelpful ways.

Keeping the interview moving

Although an assessment should have a drive towards seeking solutions and has much therapeutic value in itself, it is still using time to elicit information. Because of this, an important skill lies in knowing what information is likely to be important and how to keep the interview moving without the person feeling you are trivialising their experience, are disinterested or simply following your own agenda. Ways of attempting to keep the interview moving in a positive sense, having already conveyed the purpose of the meeting and how much time you are able to devote to it, are:

- find out what the patient wants and why;
- align yourself with the patient's agenda, i.e. concern yourself with what is important to them and what they want (without colluding with anything unhealthy or unhelpful or making promises you are not in a position to keep);
- keep the process, and your language, simple;
- avoid jargon and 'psychiatric-speak', e.g. 'your levels of observation are...' or 'I am going to be your keyworker';
- allow some digression but always bring it back to the subject that is central to your meeting – completing the assessment;
- having established clarity about your own boundaries, maintain them.

Most importantly, particular to this person and their presentation, decide what you must try and elicit and prioritise according to the circumstances and the time available.

Key clinical tip

There may be very distressing incidents or issues which the patient has difficulty discussing. If there is an issue which you think is too difficult for the person to address at any stage of the assessment, or which might take so much time it could 'derail' the assessment process, you can note it for yourself and move the assessment on, deciding as you progress whether or not to re-introduce it at a later stage in the conversation and how to do so.

Other interview techniques

Any interview requires different types of questions, differing techniques and approaches appropriate to the stage of the interview, what is being discussed and the dynamic changes in the relationship between the interviewer and interviewee. This is certainly true of a risk assessment with someone experiencing mental distress who is potentially suicidal and/or violent.

Preparing for, and during, an assessment, the assessor is continually thinking about how to ask questions, which questions to ask and when. Indeed, Albert Einstein once famously said, 'if I had an hour to solve a problem and my life depended on it, I would use the first 55 minutes determining the proper questions to ask'. This process within the assessment will also be shaped by the use of any structured risk assessment tool. As stated above, however, perhaps the best approach is to have a clear understanding of the structure of a risk assessment, the information you need to elicit and then wrap that around the story the person provides. This makes the assessment more conversational, with questions flowing from previous answers.

If the person is not answering, talking tangentially, talking over you or doesn't seem to be making sense in their replies, don't panic and think you're not completing your assessment. This is *part* of the assessment and is all valuable information that will feed into your formulation and risk management plan, e.g. if it looks as if the person is experiencing delusional beliefs or auditory hallucinations. If the person is unwilling to discuss issues related to potential risk, gently confronting that might open up the subject or, at least, offer some insight into the person's thinking. It should always be remembered that not having definitive information about risk does not mean there is no risk.

Socratic questioning

Clarke and Egan (2015) define Socratic questioning as a series of open-ended questions that encourage reflection and it is most associated with cognitive behavioural therapy. However, there is not one definition of it as a technique and, in fact, it is used in different ways in different therapies and therapeutic approaches (Carey and Mullan, 2004). In the context of risk assessment and risk management it can be employed in ways that aim to be educative, helping the person to be their own 'therapist' by helping them identify, evaluate and respond to dysfunctional thoughts and beliefs and, through that, mood and behaviour that places them at risk. Questions are used to:

- help clarify ideas or concepts and look at the rationale and evidence for these;
- explore perspectives and possible assumptions;
- help the person reflect on the implications and consequences of their thinking and decisions.

As we have seen, when people are distressed, their thoughts are often negative, distorted and unhelpful, e.g. "Nothing can help me", "I should be doing better than I am," "This is all my fault." These negative thoughts can prevent the person from seeing things as they really are, e.g. someone who is loved by their family thinking, "I'm a burden to everyone. They'd be better off without me," "They wish I was out of the way."

They can also stop the person from reaching out or learning anything new, e.g. "I don't deserve any help," and "There's no point going to see anyone. It won't be any use." These can be accompanied by dysfunctional beliefs about the self about which the person is often unaware and which are often not clearly verbalised, such as: "I'm no good," "I can't trust anyone," "No one really cares."

These are cues which the interviewer needs to listen carefully for. They may operate outside the individual's awareness and the person may be unaware of their impact. You may also hear the person articulate automatic negative thoughts, finding they spontaneously flow through their mind in the moment. For example:

- "The medication might work for other people but I'm bound to get terrible side effects."
- "No, I don't think you can help me. No one can…This is never going to change."
- "I could talk to my partner but I don't think she really wants to hear about my problems."

Individuals may or may not be aware of their automatic thoughts, but most can learn to be aware of them fairly easily. In highlighting this, the clinician:

- stimulates the person's awareness;
- focuses on defining the problem;

- exposes their belief system;
- challenges irrational beliefs while revealing the person's cognitive processes and how it relates to their risk behaviours.

Below are a range of Socratic techniques as well as other interview skills that can be used in the assessment process. Cultivating the ability to adapt, improvise and use different types of questions in response to something important mentioned by the person being assessed is important, especially if the person is finding the assessment more difficult than you'd perhaps expected.

Despite the views of some textbooks, there is not a 'perfect order' in which to use particular types of questions. Working out which question to use, and when, is as much a part of the 'live' assessment as anything.

Thus, open questions are usually the best way to start to elicit information and gain a better understanding of what it is like from the person's perspective, as they have the space to explore different themes in response to a non-specific question e.g. "How are you feeling?"

Sometimes, however, asking closed questions can prove more helpful. For someone distressed, withdrawn, overwhelmed or pre-occupied it can be difficult to respond to a request to describe their broad feelings but much easier to formulate an answer to a simpler question, e.g. "Have you been able to sleep at night over the past two weeks?"

Once the interview is flowing, it would be normal to move from open questions to 'funnelling in', to closed, specific questions, using a number of techniques to support this process. Below are types of questions and techniques you might use, with clinical examples.

Phrasing the question

What to ask, and when, can be crucial.

- Be specific when necessary – and there will be times in the interview when it is necessary, especially when stating your concerns and understanding of the risk.
- Avoid ambiguity.
- Keep your questions brief and simple.
- Allow short silences, even if you feel uncomfortable doing so – they give the patient (and yourself) time to think and respond.

Open, non-specific questions

These are best used initially e.g. "How do you feel?", "What has been happening?" or "Tell me about yourself..." Gradually, some focus can then be added e.g. "Tell me more about when you feel hopeless," or "Are there times when you don't feel like that?"

Closed questions

These elicit 'yes', 'no' or 'don't know' as an answer and can be used to provide an explicit focus and facilitate specific responses to areas of assessment where it is required. These are necessary when particular, specific information is required. Examples are: "Do you still feel like harming yourself?" or "Did you want to die when you took the tablets?" If the response is, "I don't know," or "I'm not sure," further probing is obviously required.

Funnelling in

This is crucial in building on the information that has been gained in the interview from open and non-specific questions. There will be key points you want to focus on but this should be done gradually, using each question to bring you closer to the specifics of the main area of risk to the patient.

Clinical Example 3:   Funnelling in

Clinician:	You said you were feeling desperate. Can you tell me more about that?
William:	I'd had enough. Kelly had left. Everything had gone wrong.
Clinician:	What had gone wrong?
William:	Everything. There was my dad's death… I just felt like I couldn't carry on anymore.
Clinician:	What did you do then?
William:	I got the tablets.
Clinician:	You said how you were feeling. What were you thinking?
William:	Thinking? I don't know… That it wasn't fair. That I should do something.
Clinician:	Is that something you often think? That it isn't fair?
William:	[*Silence*]
Clinician:	You said you were thinking things weren't fair and that you should do something. What did you think you should do?
William:	I… I couldn't face life anymore.
Clinician:	And?
William:	[*Pause*] I thought about ending it.
Clinician:	Ending your life?
William:	Yeah.
Clinician:	Had you thought about how you might do that?
William:	Um, yes.
Clinician:	What was your plan?
William:	To go to the station and throw myself under a train.
Clinician:	Was there a reason you thought about that particularly?
William:	How do you mean?
Clinician:	Well, I was wondering why you would think specifically of throwing yourself under a train. Had you thought about other ways in which to kill yourself but then decided against them?
William:	I took tablets before but that hadn't worked. That's why I started thinking about a train. I know there are fast trains that come through the station and… and that would be it.
Clinician:	That sounds very definite. What stopped you following through on your plan?
William:	I'm not sure. I did go down there, once, then came home. I was thinking about the driver of the train, you know, what it would be like… And I started thinking about my family having to see me…

> I just reached the stage where I couldn't think anymore. I was back home, the tablets were there. I just took them.
>
> Clinician: So, although you took them on the spur of the moment, you'd definitely been thinking about it and had something of a plan?
>
> William: Yes.

Seeking clarification

It is easy to think we understand the person's perspective or that we understand the motivation for risk behaviours without checking this out. The pattern of behaviour that led to it might appear obvious and fit within a clearly established pattern. For example, looking in from outside we see:

- the person's contact with mental health services diminishes;
- having been 'well' for a while, they question the need for prescribed medication and take it less regularly;
- an increase in stress leads to poor sleep and pronounced social anxiety;
- they attempt to self medicate using illicit drugs;
- psychotic symptoms worsen and risk behaviours occur.

However, what is important in an assessment is to go on a journey with the person and understand how they understand their situation, what they see as the problems and the precipitants. While this applies to the entire thrust of the interview it is crucial in the detail of the discussion. Seeking clarification is, therefore, an ideal opportunity to see whether or not you have understood what has been said to date, display active listening and continue to build a rapport.

Clinical Example 4:   Seeking clarification

William: It's not their fault. But no one really cares.

Clinician: Who do you mean, when you say 'no one'?

William: I don't know. Everyone. They'd be better off without me.

Clinician: Do you mean Kelly, your mum and brother?

William: Yeah. It's not their fault. I don't blame them. I'm just such a… I drag everyone down.

Clinician: How do you know that?

William: I just do.

Clinician: Have they said that to you?

William: I can see it in their faces.

Clinician: But earlier on you were telling me how worried they have been about you.

William: Yeah, but now, it's different.

Clinician: In what way? How have things changed?

William: I'm a failure.
Clinician: That's what *you* think?
William: Yeah.
Clinician: How is that connected with what you see in their faces?
William: I don't know. It's like...I just know.
Clinician: Do they do anything that shows they don't care?
William: Um, no.
Clinician: Do you think it could be anything to do with how you feel about yourself?
William: How do you mean?
Clinician: You said you feel like you're a failure. You think they'd be better off without you. Is it possible you think they think like that because that's how you feel?
William: Well...maybe... It could have been.
Clinician: But those were the thoughts running through your mind when you took the tablets?
William: Yes. And that I couldn't take anymore. I'd had enough.

When talking about risk, it is always important to be as specific as possible and if there is any doubt to seek clarification.

Clinical Example 5:   Seeking clarification

Clinician: And you said earlier you thought the tablets you took would kill you.
William: Yes.
Clinician: And a few times you've said that you wanted to escape. As I understand it, you were referring to wanting to escape the situation you'd found yourself in. Is that right?
William: And the feelings. I felt like my head was going to explode, like my whole body was on fire. And there was no way out, you know?
Clinician: Well, I'm not quite sure. This may sound a silly question, but I want to be clear that I do understand. Did you want to die? Or was dying the only way out, the only way to escape, that you could see?
William: Yeah. There is no other way out. That's obvious.
Clinician: So it isn't actually that you want to die. You want to escape.
William: Yeah. Well, both. But I had to escape from that situation.
Clinician: Let me put it another way, if there were something that would get you out of the situation and help you feel 'better', that didn't mean you had to die, would you want that?
William: Yes. [*Pause*] But there's not, is there?
Clinician: I know it doesn't feel like that for you now but I think there is.

Reflection

Occasionally, it may be useful to reflect back to the person a comment they've made, because you feel it is important and want to emphasise this, that you want to 'pause' the progress of the interview to get more information about the point that has arisen or make an empathic comment. Often, reflection is validating for the person.

Clinical Example 6:   Reflection

6.1 Simple reflection

William:	There's just times when I've completely had enough.
Clinician:	Had enough?
William:	You know, like when Kelly left. After everything else that's happened I knew I wouldn't be able to cope with that and I started thinking about killing myself.

6.2 Reflecting and gentle challenging

William:	...and everything goes wrong and there's no point because whatever I do... well...
Clinician:	Everything goes wrong?
William:	Yeah. Absolutely.
Clinician:	Yet when we were talking earlier you spoke about how you'd been able to help Kelly – and your mum and brother – with a lot of things. I've got that right, haven't I?
William:	Maybe. It doesn't feel like that now though.
Clinician:	Well, that's it, isn't it? It doesn't feel like it now but, actually, you were doing those things right up until recently.

Getting no response

If you don't get a response or the interview seems to be 'stuck' it is useful to reflect on what has happened.

- Was the question too threatening?
- Did the patient understand the question?
- Was it the 'right' question for that stage of the interview?
- Options are to:
  - re-phrase the question;
  - gently 'nudge' the patient;
  - leave it and return to it later.

If the person doesn't respond, you should directly address this rather than ignore it.

Clinical Example 7:   No response from the patient

7.1 Leave it and return later:

Clinician: You don't seem comfortable with this issue.
William: No, I'm not.
Clinician: Would you rather we come back to it later?
William: Yes.

7.2 Re-phrasing:

Clinician: You said you still feel like you can't go on. What does that mean?
William: [*Silence*]
Clinician: Has anything changed for you since you took the overdose?
William: No.
Clinician: So you still feel like killing yourself?
William: Maybe.

7.3 Gently 'nudging':

Clinician: You said you still feel like you can't go on. What does that mean?
William: [*Silence*]
Clinician: I get the sense this is a difficult subject for you, but I think it would
              be helpful for both you and me if we can try and understand how
              you're feeling now.

Confronting

Sometimes, a clinician has to be even more forthright. Often this involves making an observation. Wherever possible, you should convey the view of the clinical team but, at the same time 'own' the response with an 'I' message, so that it is clear to the person that talking to you has value and that they are clear about your views (see clinical example 8.2).

Clinical Example 8:   Confronting in a therapeutic manner

Example 8.1:

Clinician: You're telling me everything's okay and that I should let you leave
              the ward for a while, but, William, looking at you now, it doesn't
              seem as if much has changed from when you came in yesterday.
              You look as if you're feeling very distressed and I get the impression
              you're still feeling very low.

Example 8.2:

Clinician: I know you want to leave but, I'm sorry, I don't feel it would be safe to let you. It's not just me. The whole team have been very concerned about you. But I have to make a decision just now and I'd like you to remain on the ward.

Bringing a solution focused approach

Even in an assessment with an individual apparently in the midst of a terrible crisis, beset by problems, it is possible to explore solutions. This should not be confused with solution focused therapy and the solution focused assessment that is undertaken as part of this model. However, simple questions, once the degree of the problem(s) has been ascertained, allow the person to think about their earlier coping mechanism, problem solving techniques and psychological strengths.

Clinical Example 9:   A solution focused approach

Example 9.1:

William: I don't think anyone can understand what this is like. I'm never going to be able to sort any of it out. It's such a mess.
Clinician: This is obviously really difficult for you. But has anything helped you in the past when you've felt like this?

Example 9.2:

William: What am I going to do? I've failed at everything I've tried to do and I'm not surprised Kelly had enough and went. I'm useless.
Clinician: Given all that's happened, with your father dying, losing your job, Kelly and you splitting up, I think you did remarkably well to cope as well as you have up until now. How did you do that?

It is important that you are able to communicate clearly that you are not minimising the person's perception of their difficulties. Also, it needs to be remembered that someone who is depressed and suicidal will find problem solving extremely difficult, not just with practical matters but also when it comes to looking forward, to relationship issues and dealing with more abstract things, and will need to be guided through the process of how to do this.

Closing difficult issues down during the interview

There will be times when you do not want to explore an issue that comes up in an assessment. This might be for a number of reasons but is particularly useful in situations such as triage or similar, brief and focused interviews that are time limited. It may be:

- you do not think you have the expertise to do so;
- you may decide it is going to take you too far from the core issues of risk you need to assess within a given time;
- you may be concerned that exploring it now, within the context of the assessment, will lead to the person becoming too aroused and distressed, possibly jeopardising the opportunity to complete the assessment.

There are a number of ways in which you can 'close down' the issue while still communicating a number of important issues by making it clear:

- that you have 'heard' something important the person wants to tell you;
- that you do not think this is the right time to discuss it – and why:
- what you are going to do about this.

Clinical Example 10:   Closing down

Example 10.1: Discussing the issue and then drawing it to a close

Clinician: You've said that there have been times in the past you cut yourself and used other means of hurting yourself. When was the first time you did that?

William: I was about eleven...

Clinician: Can you remember what happened that you did that?

William: [*Becomes tearful*] I've never...spoken about this before.

[*Pause*]

William: My uncle had come over and... He was my dad's brother. He'd been kicked out by his wife – I guess we know why now – and... Mum and Dad went out one night, not soon after he arrived. He came in my room [*becomes tearful again*]. He did things... [*Pause*]

Clinician: Sexual things?

William: Yes.

Clinician: Was that the only time?

William: No. He did it twice more.

Clinician: Were you able to tell anyone at the time?

William: No. I didn't know what to do. I wanted to but... I was scared. I thought I'd get into trouble. Everyone felt sorry for him. It... I... You must think I'm a complete coward.

Clinician: Why do you say that?

William: Because I didn't do anything to stop him or tell anyone.

Clinician: I think you were an eleven-year-old boy in what must have been a terrifying and very confusing situation.

William: [*Silence*]

Clinician: This is obviously very important and very sensitive. And I appreciate you telling me now. It's something I think we should think about carefully. I don't want to ignore it but, because we have to finish fairly soon, I'd like to move on to talk about what happened last night, when you took the tablets. If you want to talk more about these issues, we can agree a time and talk about it later rather than try and squeeze it in now and not be able to give it the time it needs. Would that be okay with you?

William: Yeah. That's... um, well, yeah.

Clinician: So long as you feel comfortable about it. I don't want you to feel under any pressure but, when you're ready, we'll make sure we have the time.

William: Thanks. I appreciate that.

Example 10.2: An issue arises and the clinician doesn't feel fully competent to address it

William: That was when... when things started to happen, when my uncle came into the house and I was on my own.

Clinician: I understand it might be important for you to talk about this but, to be honest, it's not an area in which I have a lot of experience. I'm going to ask one of my colleagues if they can talk more with you about this later. It's not that I don't want to help, but I think you'd benefit more from talking with someone who has more experience.

Example 10.3: An issue arises which might deter from a key moment in the risk assessment

William: It's like when I start thinking about stuff... about things that happened when my uncle came into the house... when my mum and dad weren't there...

Clinician: This is obviously distressing for you. I also get the sense that it's important but I think it would be better if, right now, we stay focused on what was happening when you decided to take the tablets and then return to it after, if you feel okay about that. I'll make sure we have time to talk about it a bit later. Is that okay?

William: We'll definitely talk about it? Now I've spoken about it... you know.

Clinician: Definitely. I hear how important it is.

William: Okay. Thanks.

Digression

As noted above, while having an internalised assessment structure, knowledge of what information you are seeking and what types of questions and interview techniques to use at different stages of the assessment, it is a high level skill to be able to facilitate the person digressing while being able to bring it back to the core issues with the assessment. In Clinical Example 11, using Oliver's case study (see Box 2), we see the clinician exploring further elements of his psychotic thinking before returning to the central theme of exploring a recent assault on another patient.

In this example, the clinician digresses from asking solely about why Oliver has hit fellow patient Daniel to explore something about his psychotic experiences and validate his distress, while not colluding with his beliefs or condoning Oliver's violent behaviour.

Clinical Example 11: Digression

Clinician: So it was when you thought Daniel did something to you that you decided you would hit him?

Oliver: I didn't just think it. You're like all the others. You reckon this is all in my head.

Clinician: I'm sorry. I didn't mean to convey that impression at all. Could you tell me what happened?

Oliver: He's been at it for ages and you all let him. You don't care.

Clinician: What had he been doing? Could you explain?

Oliver: No. Why should I?

Clinician: {Silence]

Oliver: He's been trying to infect me, hasn't he? Like you lot.

Clinician: Us lot?

Oliver: You know. Some of the nurses do it as well.

Clinician: Try to infect you?

Oliver: Yeah.

Clinician: How does that work?

Oliver: Putting their thoughts into me. Wanting me to do things. Take my powers away.

Clinician: What powers?

Oliver: You know.

Clinician: I'm sorry, Oliver. I'm not being difficult. I honestly don't know.

Oliver: Well, you should know.

Clinician: Like I said, I'm sorry. Sometimes I'm a bit slow. It would help me if you told me.

Oliver: It's obvious, ain't it? Like, my strength. My thoughts. My mind.

Clinician: What's the reason Daniel and these nurses do that?

Oliver: Because they're scared of me, of course.

Clinician: What are they scared of? Something you could do?

Oliver: Just my powers. I can do anything if I want. They think I'd hurt them. But I wouldn't. Not unless they start attacking me like Daniel did.

Clinician: Do you know how they do this? The infecting, I mean.

Oliver: No, not really. It's like they do it with their thoughts.

Clinician: So how do you know when it's happening?

Oliver: 'Cause I can feel it. My heart starts going a bit faster. Things start happening in my gut. I feel like something's been put in my legs, like

> I can't stand still but my feet go funny, spongy like. I can't think straight. My thoughts are all fuzzy, like.
>
> Clinician: That sounds awful.
> Oliver: Yeah. It is.
> Clinician: Was that happening just before you hit Daniel?
> William: Yeah.
> Clinician: And was that why you hit him, or was it because of the cigarettes?
> Oliver: I'm not worried about the cigarettes. I could've got those back. It did annoy me a bit and I might have given him a slap about that. But it was this infecting thing. I'm not having it, am I?

Summarising

During the course of a risk assessment it is often useful to pause to reflect on what information has emerged and how you have understood it.

Remembering that the person's cognitive functioning is likely to be impaired by anxiety and psychological arousal, it provides an opportunity to remind them of what has been said up until that point. It also allows you to:

* state the key points as you've understood them from the discussion so far;
* check if your understanding matches that of the patient;
* see if you have missed anything;
* check if the person wants to add anything;
* discuss what comes next, given the point reached at this stage of the interview.

Clinical Example 12: Summarising

Clinician: It might be useful if we pause for a moment to summarise where we have got to. As I understand it, from what you've said, this has been a very difficult few months, with pressures at work, your father's death. You weren't sleeping well, your concentration was poor and you were feeling low in mood, as well as having panic attacks. You lost your job unexpectedly. Then Kelly left and that was the last straw. It was then you started to think about killing yourself. Is that right?

William: Kind of. Things hadn't been right between me and Kelly for a while. I was feeling sorry for myself and I was taking it out on her. And I think I was maybe drinking a bit too much sometimes. Not much. But sometimes. I know Kelly didn't like it.

Clinician: I think I missed that. My apologies. It's useful and maybe we'll come back to it a bit later? Is there anything else I've missed, or is there anything I should have asked you about?

William: No. That's about it.
Clinician: All right.

Towards the end of any assessment, ask yourself, what don't I know? Is there anything that's been said that I don't understand? Do I think there are any gaps in the story? Do I understand how this person got to this point? Is there anything about the risks about which I'm unsure? If there is, you have the opportunity to explore it while the person is with you.

Genuineness

If you can utilise the skills outlined above and combine them with something of your own personality, this can be very useful in helping with your rapport and moving the risk assessment process forward. Stuart (2005) has described genuineness in the nurse-patient relationship as 'the nurse is an open, honest and sincere person who is actively involved in the relationship'. This is achieved by the nurse thinking and feeling the same thing, not suppressing feelings and, most importantly, saying the same thing(s) as they are thinking and feeling.

To this, perhaps, can be added something else. In focusing on the person being assessed and what they are saying, being mindful of that person, you are more likely to respond to them rather than thinking about what you 'should' say in the circumstances. Undoubtedly, this is partly about confidence, which in turn comes from having experience and knowing something about how you cope under pressure. It is also about feeling confident enough to bring something of your own personality into the process, to know when and how much it is appropriate to self disclose, using your own 'voice' while remembering that you are also trying to tap into the language of the person you're assessing.

Over time this will help you find your own way of expressing clinical terminology, so 'keyworker' might become 'the person who'll be working with you', a 'care plan' might be called 'an agreement between us about the work we'll be doing' and an 'assessment' a 'discussion between us where I'll be asking lots of questions so we can try and figure out, together, what's been happening'.

Concreteness

This is an essential communications tool used in developing and maintaining therapeutic relationships. In the context of risk assessment it involves being specific, particularly when discussing the patient's feelings, experiences and behaviours. It 'avoids vagueness and ambiguity and is the opposite of generalising, labelling, and making assumptions about the patient's experience', all essential in formulating a good risk assessment (Stuart, 2005).

Respect

Respect encompasses politeness, aspects of empathy and genuineness. Although it may seem a very simple thing, and something that is trotted out in many nursing texts, to be respectful of someone who behaves in a very challenging manner or who has done things that go against your own ethical or moral codes is never easy. It involves accepting the person for who they are, being able to listen to, and accept, their story neutrally, with curiosity and without exhibiting judgement or criticism, no matter what you're thinking or feeling. Behaviours, feelings and attitudes are accepted as unique to that person given the circumstances in which they found themselves.

The importance of respect in assessing and managing risk is that it both acknowledges the potential for change as and when circumstances are different and makes it easier for the person to tell their story, particularly those parts of it that have been very distressing and/or disturbing.

A clinician displaying personal attributes such as respect and politeness may also make it easier for the person to accept things from the clinician that might otherwise provoke a more challenging reaction.

Self disclosure

This can be another tool for helping you build a relationship with the person you are assessing. Knowing what and how much to disclose is never easy but should reflect a genuine, respectful and empathic relationship with the person and have a therapeutic purpose e.g. to model something, be educative, validate feelings or develop the therapeutic alliance you are attempting to foster.

Different clinical services will have different approaches and even rules about this. In prisons and forensic settings, for example, there will be strict rules governing self disclosure, where the nature of the risk can be very different. Knowing the policy on this is essential, as is consistency, genuineness and honesty (see clinical example 13.2).

Clinical Example 13:   Self disclosure

Example 13.1: In a community mental health setting

Clinician:	So things between Kelly and yourself were difficult for a while?
William:	Yes. [*Pause, looking at the wedding ring on the clinician's hand*] Are you married?
Clinician:	Yes, I've been married for several years.
William:	But you wear your ring on your right hand.
Clinician:	I broke my finger a few years ago and the joint swells, so I can't put it on anymore. Why do you ask?
William:	I don't know. You look the type to be married.
Clinician:	Are you wondering if I can understand your situation?
William:	I doubt you've got a relationship like I had with Kelly.
Clinician:	Tell me about your relationship with Kelly then, perhaps, I can understand.

Example 13.2: In a forensic setting

Clinician:	So you were brought up in Scotland but then moved to London?
Oliver:	Yeah. Where do you live?
Clinician:	I'm sorry, Oliver. There are rules about what we're allowed to tell people here and that's not something I can discuss.
Oliver:	I only asked where you live, mate. It's not like I'm going 'round there, is it?
Clinician:	A lot of people are curious about things like that and can be frustrated by the answer but, as I said, I'm sorry, there are rules and I can't discuss it. Why were you interested?

Oliver:	Well. You're asking me a lot of questions. I just thought... I dunno.
Clinician:	There are other ways in which we can get to know each other, even with those constraints.
Oliver:	Like what?
Clinician:	Let's see how we go, eh? So what was it like, coming from a village in Scotland to London?
Oliver:	I hated it.

In the first example the clinician notes William looking at his wedding ring and doesn't avoid the question but, without revealing anything other than he's married, uses it as an opportunity to explore William's feelings, not only about his relationship with his own partner but also how much he feels understood in the assessment.

In the second example, the clinician is honest and to the point, explaining that there are rules and they are following them. When challenged about this, the answer remains the same, courteous, acknowledging that others might share that curiosity and the potential frustration at not receiving an answer before trying to move the discussion on.

Things to avoid

Avoid leading questions

Leading questions and assumptions can cause all sorts of problems. If the information has not yet been established, e.g. whether or not the person actually intended to kill himself, asking, "Why did you want to kill yourself?" reveals an assumption on the part of the questioner and also closes off a whole range of issues.

Instead, ask: "When you took the tablets, what was your intention?"

If the answer is still not clear, you can ask a closed question: "Did you want to kill yourself?"

Avoid multiple questions

For example, "Do you have trouble getting off to sleep or wake up early? What do you think about when you can't sleep?" This is actually three separate questions.

Instead, separate the questions and ask them one at a time:

1. "Do you have trouble getting off to sleep?"
2. "Do you wake up early?"
3. "What do you think about when you can't sleep?"

Avoid failing to validate the person's experience

This is quite difficult, particularly if the person you are assessing is psychotic, and requires some thought when responding to the person's story as they explain it.

Clinical Example 14: Not validating the person's experience

Clinician: Tell me more about these ideas you get about Daniel and others infecting you.

Oliver: You're like all the others. You don't believe me. They're not ideas. It's real. There's no point talking to you.

Clinician: I just want to know more about why you started threatening people.

Oliver: I wasn't threatening anyone. I'm going.

Such a situation as that in Clinical Example 14 (above) can potentially be avoided by adopting a different way of exploring the issue.

Clinical Example 15: Validating the person's experience

Clinician: Tell me more about what happened between you and Daniel.

Oliver: What, the infecting thing?

Clinician: Yes.

Oliver: He does it to wind me up and because he's scared of me.

Clinician: And do you get wound up?

Oliver: Of course. Anyone would.

Clinician: What happens to you when you're wound up?

Oliver: I have to do things.

Clinician: What sort of things?

Oliver: I don't know... I have to get rid of the feeling. What it's like. Being wound up.

Clinician: What does it feel like?

Oliver: It's horrible. Like everything inside me is rigid and there's loads of energy buzzing through me but my head's full of stuff and I can't think. I feel all sweaty and I just want them to stop it.

Clinician: It does sound horrible, a bit like things feeling out of control.

Oliver: Exactly.

In this example, the clinician hasn't colluded with Oliver's belief that other patients can 'infect' him and that is the source of his psychological and physiological state of arousal. But by asking Oliver more about what he believes to be happening and then validating Oliver's feelings related to his experience, he is able to elicit crucial information that progresses his risk assessment, particularly in relation to Oliver feeling threatened and that things are out of his control.

Closing, or finishing, the assessment interview

This is a vital part of the interview when you will seek to summarise and consolidate all that you have discussed in your time with the patient. It should incorporate a discussion about the key issues that have arisen, including risks, an attempt to understand the context of these risks (very similar to a clinical formulation but in the individual's own language) and move onto a plan for future contact and risk management (see Table 3.3).

Clinical Example 16:   Closing the session

Clinician: Thanks for taking so much of your time to talk with me, particularly as there were some things it was clear were very upsetting.

William: Yes, well... I don't want to go through this anymore. You know, these thoughts going round in my head, the feeling like I'm going to collapse. It's too much.

Clinician: I did pick that up, very strongly, from everything you said. In fact, I just wanted to go over the key things as I understood them and make sure I haven't missed anything, is that okay?

William: Yeah.

Clinician: From what you were saying, it's been a very difficult few months, since your father's death –

William: I'd been struggling before that, when he was ill... you know, like I said...

Clinician: Yes, I was going to come to that. But it seems as if you felt much worse after his death, less able to cope with the sort of things you'd been managing to do previously. You weren't sleeping well, you were feeling low, couldn't concentrate, then lost your job and money problems mounted up. Is that right?

William: Yeah, and then Kelly...

Clinician: And after Kelly left you began having more thoughts about suicide, and then took the tablets with the intention of killing yourself?

William: [*Looks down at the floor and nods*]

Clinician: But this had been building for a long time–

William: My whole life, it seems now.

Clinician: Yes, you were saying it had brought up a lot of stuff from when you were very young, as well as your first marriage and things you've struggled with for a long time. Including your uncle abusing you.

William: [*Looks up, becomes slightly tearful but nods again*]

Clinician: So we've agreed that, because you're still having very strong thoughts about killing yourself and don't feel able to resist them, particularly if you're back at the flat on your own and even with people coming in to see you, you'll come into hospital for a short period of time while we look at how we can help you look at other options. I'll talk to the doctor about starting that antidepressant we discussed but also think about how to help you look again at some of the problems you've identified.

William: I can't really think much more. I feel exhausted.

Clinician:	You look very tired. While we arrange to take you into hospital I'm going to get you a drink and sandwich if you'd like one. I'll also give you a copy of that plan, or agreement, we talked about so you can have a look at it. But only when you're ready. There's no rush. It lists the things we'll do to try and help, as I explained, as well as the things you thought you could do. I'll also get the leaflets about the ward and medication. I know it's a lot, and I don't expect you to take it all in just now. It will be there so you can look at them in your own time when you've had a chance to rest a bit. Is there anything I've missed? Anything else you need to tell me before we finish?
William:	No.
Clinician:	Good.

Table 3.3 Closing the session – key points

- Summarise the content of the interview.
- Summarise what has been agreed.
- Particularly focus on any risk management plan.
- Who will do what, e.g. patient and clinician to 'manage' risks.
- Ensure the person has nothing else to ask or clarify.
- Provide a reminder of what will happen with information, e.g. documentation.
- Agree what will happen next, e.g. next appointment or meeting.

Risk assessment in the context of a full mental health assessment

So far, we have explored interviewing someone either already well known to you or your service where the key requirement is a risk assessment in the context of the person's current circumstances. The structure of this interview is relatively straightforward: 'what happened, what was the person thinking/feeling, what did the person want to happen' etc. However, there are times when a risk assessment, or re-assessment, is required as part of a full mental health assessment. An example would be when meeting someone not previously known to you or the service.

It could also include someone who has not been assessed for a period during which there could have been significant changes, perhaps due to the time since they were last assessed or simply something about how the person now sees their experience.

There are numerous ways in which to construct a mental health assessment and, in part, these might be defined by the use of specific assessment tools, e.g. KGV-M Assessment Tool, The Carers and Users Expectation of Services (CUES), Beck's Depression Inventory, Liverpool University Neuroleptic Side Effects Rating Scale (LUNSERS), while there are also tools that can be used to assist the risk assessment process, including the Galatean Risk Screening Tool (GRIST), Historical Clinical Risk-20 (HCR-20), Short Term Assessment of Risk and Treatability (START), Sexual Violence Risk-20 (SVR-20) and Violence Risk Appraisal Guide (VRAG).

When using any assessment tool, think about what is *not* contained within its questions. The tool should never be used as a 'checklist' or thought to contain the framework that will necessarily give you the answers you need. It will provide answers to the questions contained in it but you may need to ask completely different questions, picking up on cues and issues arising out of the assessment, to give you as full as possible an understanding of the risk to the person and/or others.

However, while the risk assessment essentially remains the same, there are a wide number of ways in which it can be placed within the interview process. This guide suggests a structure that aims to build a full picture of the individual and all aspects of their history before addressing risk as a specific issue, thus beginning with 'the history of the presenting complaint' and ending with risk.

There are obviously huge numbers of texts that offer advice and the evidence base for undertaking a mental health assessment and mental state examination. The *Pocket Guide* is not going to replicate these but focus on different components of the assessment as they *potentially* relate to risk, particularly to the individual being assessed and/or others but also exploring vulnerability in the context of a deteriorating mental state. To assist in this, a character called Emma will be used as the case study. Unlike William and Oliver, the details of her character and background will be revealed through the assessment process.

Appearance and behaviour

As stressed throughout the *Pocket Guide*, what you see is very important, particularly in terms of congruence, and the first part of a mental state examination is actually to note how the person appears and behaves during the interview. Particularly, thinking of motivation and a willingness to collaborate with the process of risk management:

- Does the person volunteer information, are they elusive or find it difficult to articulate their experience?
- Is there anything to indicate the person's level of self care, e.g. have they washed, are their clothes clean or is their hair unwashed etc?
- How are they dressed?
- What is the person's facial expression?
- Have they any distinctive marks, scars, tattoos etc?
- What is the person's emotional and cognitive state *during* the interview? Does it vary? Is there anything particular that is distressing for them? Does the person appear distracted, pre-occupied etc?
- Are they restless?
- Do their reactions and responses seem appropriate, in your opinion, to the situation (and it is important to stress that this area of assessment is highly subjective)?

History of presenting complaint

This involves identifying the background to issues leading to the current presentation. The approach is partly determined by the circumstances that led to the person and how they came to be seeing you now, and particularly the urgency of the consultation. Did they:

- Seek help themselves?
- Have to be encouraged to seek help?
- Get brought in by the police/carers/others and are unwilling to be with you now?

However, to establish clarity, it's important to set some parameters, e.g. "Tell me what brought you here now."

The key words are: 'here' and 'now'.

Clinical Example 17: Focusing on the immediate reasons the person is being assessed

Clinician:	Tell me what brought you here now.
Emma:	Well, I'm feeling pretty depressed.
Clinician:	I'm sorry to hear that. How long have you been feeling like that?
Emma:	I don't know. Years. Most of my life really.
Clinician:	Okay. What was different that you came here today?
Emma:	I haven't been able to sleep. I'm feeling a lot more anxious… It feels like it's getting worse.
Clinician:	What has changed in the last few days or weeks that you've been feeling like that?

Key clinical tip

Focusing on the 'here' and 'now' at the start of the risk assessment provides focus and allows you to gain an understanding of the immediate problem(s).

Full biographical history

It is easy to assume we 'know' a person, their experience and can understand what is happening with them, particularly when there is a lot of documentation about that person, either in the form of reports or previous assessments. However, there may be mistakes or inaccuracies in reports that have become regarded as 'truths' about the person. Nothing can be as useful as hearing from the person about how they understand and relate their experience.

The aim of taking a biographical history is to elicit:

- Who is this person?
- How do they see themselves?
- How do the events that have brought them to you fit into their life?

Explore the details of their:

- family;
- education;
- employment;
- social circumstances;
- economic circumstances;
- relationship and sexual history.

There are obviously potentially difficult areas to negotiate here but, if the flow of the questions relates to the person's story and has progressed reasonably well, it is best to address them in a very straightforward manner (see clinical example 18).

One of the most daunting for less experienced clinicians, however, is the issue of a full psychosexual history. It can feel intrusive and not as important as other aspects of the person's life. Particularly, there may be an anxiety about sexual abuse being disclosed or, if it has in previous assessments, being spoken about. This is, nonetheless, crucial information in the area of a person's life, given the close relationship of trauma and abuse to risks such as self-harm and possible suicidal ideation. It may be, as well, that the person being assessed has been abusive in relationships. Even if abuse is absent, sex and sexual relationships are an important part of most people's lives and warrant exploration.

As is discussed later, an assessment is not a therapy session and you won't have the time to explore abuse in any depth, nor is it appropriate or helpful to bring it out into the open and then just 'leave it', so it does take some skill to ask about it and then ensure the person feels heard while being able to gently close it down with an indication of what you will do with any information divulged and how they will be helped in the future (see clinical example 10).

As with any potentially difficult areas of the assessment, building towards it helps the person, while the offer of 'opting out' of answering should remain. Thus, in exploring relationships, you start by asking about friendships, from the local area, school, university, work etc, then ask about partners and go onto sexual relationships, it gives the person being assessed some continuity and a logical progression. It also makes it easier to then move onto asking if the person feels they has ever been abused in any way, including physically, psychologically or sexually.

In conclusion, you cannot expect someone to necessarily divulge their most intimate secrets when first meeting you just because you want then to. You will have to work to develop a rapport, earn their trust and display genuine curiosity within a framework that is compassionate and concerned. A full biographical history in risk assessments helps us try to understand the idiosyncrasies and important events that have shaped the individual's life, their psyche and their attitudes to issues of risk and why they are struggling at this particular time.

In clinical example 18, Emma has presented at an emergency mental health service, having jumped from a bridge into a river the day before in an apparent suicide attempt. She has an earlier diagnosis of emotionally unstable personality disorder (EUPD), though disputes this. Her biographical history reveals a series of traumatic episodes and periods of neglect. It is a challenging interview as Emma struggles with the interview structure, as well as her own feelings and thoughts. However, we can see how her current risk is inextricably bound up with her early experiences and the clinician is able to make sense of how these are impacting on her in the moment.

Clinical Example 18:   Looking at the person's biographical history and family relationships

[*The clinician is summarising what Emma has said about why she asked to be seen now*]

Clinician: Okay, from what I understand, although you've had some serious problems for quite a few years, you're here today because

	you've been having stronger urges to cut yourself and yesterday you jumped into the river when you were thinking about killing yourself. Is that right?
Emma:	I want to die. That's what I said.
Clinician:	Yes. And this is because you've been stressed about your university course and problems have been building at home?
Emma:	My mother is a monster. That's all you need to know.
Clinician:	But I think you also said it was because you were supposed to be going out with your friends and–
Emma:	Yeah. But then, suddenly, out of nothing, it's like I don't exist. No messages. Nothing. I'm cancelled. I know they've all gone out. Why would they just drop me like that?
Clinician:	I don't know. What do you think?
Emma:	They've obviously been planning it. It's been like, "Oh, you're our best friend. We love you," all the time since starting uni but it was all a game. Ha ha. Let's all have a good laugh at Emma. I'm done with them.
Clinician:	We'll come back to all of that a bit later, if you don't mind? That's the last few days. I wanted to clarify though, were you feeling suicidal before the problems with your pals? You went to the river–
Emma:	They're not my 'pals'. Are they? And what, are you playing detective now?
Clinician:	I'm sorry. I didn't mean anything by using the work 'pals'. It's my age. And I only wanted to make sure I understand the sequence of things.
Emma:	Well, you do, okay? So can we please move on?
Clinician:	Definitely. As I said at the beginning of the interview, I want to hear from you about your past, from growing up at home all the way through to now.
Emma:	Read my notes.
Clinician:	I have had a look but, as I said earlier, I find it makes it easier if you're able to tell me in your own words about yourself.
Emma:	Half of what's written about me is lies anyway. I've seen some really useless people sitting in your chair in the past.
Clinician:	Emma, I know–
Emma:	Like, they say I have emotionally unstable personality disorder. I don't. I have complex PTSD. I was told that by a private psychiatrist last year.
Clinician:	And I think you're on a waiting list for an assessment by our complex case team. Is that right?
Emma:	Yeah. But that's taking, like, forever. I'll be dead before they even offer me an appointment. I've told them that. I rang up last week, and I said, "I'm having suicidal thoughts. I'm going to take an overdose or I'm going to jump in the river." They don't care. They said, "Go and see your keyworker. That's what she's there for."

	I haven't seen her in two months. And when I do, she just sits there, like a plank, with no idea of what to say. She's worse than useless.
Clinician:	So, there are big issues about the support that's available to you. I do recognise there have been very difficult times and I don't want you to feel pressured, so we'll go at your pace, okay?
Emma:	[*Nods*]
Clinician:	Who was at home when you were growing up?
Emma:	My mum and my dad. He was really sweet and kind but she destroyed him. She does that with everyone.
Clinician:	What happened to your dad?
Emma:	He died. He had a heart attack. My brother and I found him lying on the floor in the living room. He must have died the night before. He was all blue and discoloured.
Clinician:	This might sound like a stupid question, but what was that like for you?
Emma:	It was grotesque. I had nightmares for weeks. I still see him. There was a smell. I'll never forget it. My poor dad. Everything would have been different if he hadn't died.
[*Pause*]	
Emma:	What's wrong with you? Why don't you say something?
Clinician:	I was just thinking about what that must have been like for you. What happened after that?
Emma:	It was chaos. Mum was depressed and psychotic for about two years. Suicide attempts, staying in bed for weeks. Saying nothing for weeks then wild tantrums. Taking everything out on us – me and my brother.
Clinician:	It sounds... I don't know... I'm trying to imagine how you coped.
Emma:	Then she started drinking and never really stopped. But, you see, underneath all of that, she was a monster. She always was. That's what caused my dad's heart attack. But nobody believed it. She was the tragic widow and the upstanding geography teacher.
Clinician:	Who looked after you while your mum was ill?
Emma:	Our aunt used to stay over but she had her own family to look after. And gran was always depressed. Our aunt had to look after her as well.
Clinician:	Were social services ever involved?
Emma:	Are you joking? It was all covered up. Our family don't do scandal. We're too good for that. Then there were the 'uncles', she must have had sex with half the men in Guildford. But why should I tell you any of this? You won't do anything. I'm not going to see you again. You'll be like every other person who says they're going to help me.

Clinician:	I want to be able to help you as best I can this evening.
Emma:	Huh. So what else do you want to know? About the two 'uncles' who touched me up or the one I had an affair with when I was 13?
Clinician:	[*Pauses*] I read about this in your records. You talked a lot about this with the Child and Adolescent team–
Emma:	So you're not interested. Why ask then?
Clinician:	Why do you think I'm not interested?
Emma:	Because no one is.
Clinician:	I know talking about being abused–
Emma:	Well. I thought I was being clever in seducing him but, of course, he was rubbing his hands, grooming me all along…
Clinician:	Which is abuse. I might be wrong, but I get the impression that the way you talk about this doesn't reflect how you might feel about it. Going into it now might be very painful because it sounds as if it was very traumatic.
Emma:	[*Silence*]
Clinician:	Was it on your mind over the past few weeks?
Emma:	It's always there. And what my mum did. Everything.
Clinician:	Your mum did?
Emma:	The beatings. When she was unwell. When she was drunk.
Clinician:	And have you been thinking about all this more over the last few weeks?
Emma:	It's worse when I'm stressed and I've been, like, really stressed about how I'm going to get back to uni and get my degree.
Clinician:	With so much trauma at home, what was school like?
Emma:	It used to be my refuge.
Clinician:	Until?
Emma:	Until Steve. The guy. My mother's guy I… whatever…
Clinician:	How did that change things?
Emma:	Everyone found out. I stopped going to school – I was embarrassed – and I made friends with these other girls and started doing things, you know, that proper young ladies aren't supposed to do.
Clinician:	Such as?
Emma:	Using drugs, boys, I don't know. Everything went a bit crazy.
Clinician:	Do you know why that was?
Emma:	No, not really. I felt so bad. Everything was out of control.

[*Later in the interview, after they have finished discussing Emma's personal history, current social circumstances and mental state, the clinician summarises*]

Clinician:	At the moment, then, you've taken a year out of university, you're back with your mum, and your anxiety has got a lot worse, your mood is lower – you said it's 1/10 most of the time, with one being

	the lowest it could be – you're not sleeping well, you've been occasionally bingeing your food and drinking more alcohol–
Emma:	It sounds pathetic, doesn't it?
Clinician:	Is that what you think?
Emma:	[*Silence*]
Clinician:	It sounds to me like you've been having an incredibly difficult time. In fact, I'm surprised that, with everything that was happening, you were still able to get such good A level results and go to university. But what is really impressive is that you're getting this short story published. How do you feel about that?
Emma:	I'm hoping to get another two accepted. They're nearly finished. Maybe I'll be the Sylvia Plath of the 21st century.
Clinician:	Sylvia Plath took her own life. Do you think you'll do that?
Emma:	Probably.
Clinician:	Maybe you'll be the Margaret Attwood.
Emma:	You're showing off now.
Clinician:	That brings us to the recent ideas you've been having about cutting yourself and jumping off the bridge.
Emma:	I'm either going to be left alone and not treated like a piece of shit, so I can live a completely normal life, or I'm going to end it. That's why I'm here now, to see which way it's going to go. I'm sick of being deliberately messed around, promised help that never materialises and fobbed off.
Clinician:	There's a lot there. The idea of either being able to live a completely normal life or ending your life, that sounds very black and white. And it's a lot of pressure on the two of us, now, to sort everything out.
Emma:	So? That's your job, isn't it?
Clinician:	What is it people do that makes you think they're deliberately messing you around and fobbing you off?
Emma:	I just know. Right?
Clinician:	But, from what you've been saying, these are the things you think about, along with the memories of things from your past, that stress you out, leave you feeling depressed?
Emma:	Yes. And dearest mother. The last few days she's been even worse. Wanting me to do everything for her, constantly criticising me, then blaming me for her illness and my dad's death.
Clinician:	After she said that, was that when you left the house yesterday?
Emma:	Yes. I had no choice, if she's going to carry on like that. Plus my so called friends refusing to answer me when I was trying to get in touch.
Clinician:	Those were the triggers?
Emma:	Yes.
Clinician:	And in situations like that, is it like you said before, feeling more and more upset, sad – and angry – then thinking about ending your life?

Emma:	Yes. Everything's spiralling out of control and I have to.
Clinician:	Is that why you went to the bridge?
Emma:	I never went to the bridge to jump. I was just walking across it. And then I just thought, 'why not?'
Clinician:	You didn't plan it, or go there for that purpose?
Emma:	Nope.
Clinician:	Did you want to die when you jumped?
Emma:	I'm not sure. When I jumped in, maybe, but when those two guys pulled me out and called the ambulance, I'd calmed down. Anyway, they were really sweet and I just went home.
Clinician:	On the bus? In your wet clothes?
Emma:	Yeah. They were going to get me a taxi but no taxi driver would let me in their cab like that. Even I know that. And no one on the bus even looked at me or asked if I was okay. Very British, eh?
Clinician:	You must have been freezing.
Emma:	I just felt like a complete idiot.
Clinician:	But the thoughts didn't go away and got worse overnight, which is why you came here?
Emma:	Yes.
Clinician:	You said you were going to cut across your breasts and abdomen. Why was that?
Emma:	It usually stops the thoughts if I cut myself.
Clinician:	How would it help you to cut your breasts and abdomen?
Emma:	To make myself look ugly.
Clinician:	Is that how you feel about yourself?
Emma:	Yeah. Don't you think I'm ugly?
Clinician:	I can hear that a lot of things you might think are ugly have happened to you. How can we help you stay safe?

From the interview, Emma's strained relationship with her clinical team and mental health services is revealed, her perception of being abandoned by the team and repeatedly let down. This clearly mirrors something of her relationship with her mother. Her difficulty managing her current stress and the behaviour of her mother have, by her account, become overwhelming and she continues to struggle with memories of past trauma. The perceived sudden rejection by her university friends seems to have been the trigger for this crisis.

Emma's labile emotional state, anger and mistrust of clinicians all point to potential difficulties in helping her keep herself safe in the short term, even though she is identifying long term goals, i.e. going back to university and getting more short stories published. Given this, there is an inherent risk in basing a risk management plan on Emma collaborating consistently with clinicians in the community. At the same time, there would need to be a very clear understanding of what a community service would offer, not just post assessment but if the situation deteriorated.

> **Key clinical tip**
>
> As well as helping establish a rapport before moving onto potentially more diffi-cult topics, starting at 'the beginning' of someone's story, i.e. their family and very early background, establishes a chronological pattern to the interview, making it easier for the person to think about what is coming and feeling less 'surprised' by particular questions.

Exploring the person's health

Take a full history of any physical and mental health problems, including treatment, time(s) in hospital etc, as well as any ongoing treatment and/or contact with services.

Drugs and alcohol

This is explored historically, from the time of first using alcohol and/or substances, in-cluding the circumstances of early and ongoing drug and alcohol use, reasons for it and its impact. The drugs used should be clearly identified, how much of any drug used and frequency. Any change over time should be discussed. The discussion should not be con-fined to 'street' or illicit drugs, remembering that people can misuse prescribed or over the counter medicines and they can be equally dangerous in these circumstances.

The same should be probed for alcohol use, including patterns of drinking, during a 24-hour period and over time.

Having established any historical use of drugs and alcohol, an exploration of current usage naturally follows. Again, this should look at daily consumption, e.g. at what time it starts, how much is taken, what prompts it, when it stops and why; patterns over a weekly period, e.g. is it regular, binged, predictable, impulsive etc.; identifying reasons for any misuse, e.g. 'self medicating', peer pressure, social circumstances, pleasure etc and its impact. As always, in this context, looking at how current usage impacts on risk is key.

Particular attention should be paid to any occasions where withdrawal symptoms have been experienced, what those symptoms were and the context, i.e. what was the person's drug and/or alcohol consumption at the time, how much time would elapse be-tween consumption and withdrawal symptoms, would the person wake up in the morn-ing and already be experiencing symptoms.

Mental state examination

This is a complex and detailed area of the assessment and there is not space to explore every aspect of it. Reference to further reading is detailed below while the broad content of a mental state examination is summarised in Table 3.4.

Exploring the issues in Table 3.4 in detail is not always possible for various reasons. Perhaps it is a matter of time, perhaps the clinician given the responsibility for undertak-ing the risk assessment will not have been trained in taking a mental state examination (MSE) or have the experience. This does *not* preclude undertaking a risk assessment. Moreover, a full MSE may not be necessary.

Table 3.4 Risk and the mental state examination

Component of the MSE	What is being explored
Speech and language	• Fluency of speech (rate, volume, tone). • Pressure of speech. • Content. • Form.
Thought: form	• Degree of connectedness. • Continuity of thought. • Linearity of thought. • Formal thought disorder, e.g. loosening of association, knight's move thinking, word salad, thought block, perseveration and neologisms. • Psychic retardation. • Slowed tempo of thought. • Accelerated tempo of thought. • Flight of ideas. • Goal-directedness.
Thought: content	• Pre-occupations. • Ruminations. • Obsessions. • Topics. • Phobias. • Abnormal thoughts. • Delusions or overvalued ideas. • Thought interference, reference or persecution. • Control or passivity. • Thoughts of self-harm, suicide or homicide.
Mood (the person's emotional state over a longer period of time) **Affect** (the emotional state of the person at a given moment in time)	**Objectively**, does the person appear: • Elated? • Flat/blunted? • Incongruous? • Depressed or anxious? • Angry or irritable? • Is their mood reactive, for example do they smile when talking of something they enjoy? **Subjectively**: how does the person describe their mood? • Does this match your impression?
Perceptions **Cognitions**	• Hallucinations, other perceptual disturbance. • Attention & concentration. • Orientation to time, place and person. • Level of comprehension. • Short-term memory.
Insight (this actually means the power or act of seeing into a situation but can also be understood as how the person perceives their experience)	• How does the person understand their experience? • Do they share the same views as others about their behaviour and its causes? • Does the person see their situation as unusual and due to changes in their mental state? Do they have some awareness that they may be 'different' but have an alternative explanation for this?

However, if a formal MSE is not going to be part of the assessment process, you should nonetheless develop an understanding of how the person's mental state is impacting on potential issues of risk. For example:

- Is the person depressed – remembering depression is the mental disorder that carries the greatest risk of suicide?
- Is the person psychotic – is their psychotic experience influencing their behaviour in a potentially dangerous way?

Current circumstances

Having looked at past history and circumstances and current mental state, an exploration of the person's current circumstances is necessary, focusing on how this may impact on risk. It should encompass:

- housing – where they live, if temporary, rented or being purchased, who lives with them; social support in the form of family and/or carers, friends, ongoing relationships, the nature and quality of those relationships;
- employment and finances – are they working, what their job is, have they any financial concerns;
- if younger, are they in permanent education, e.g. at school, university or studying. Is this impacting on their mental health and potential risk behaviours?
- Religious and/or spiritual views and how these might impact on risk behaviours.

From all of this, it should be easier to then examine risk and understand how any feelings and ideas the person has about risk and risk behaviours fit into this person's life, current mental, psychological and emotional state. Static and dynamic risk factors will have emerged. Risk factors will have either been hinted at or, in some cases, clarified. Any risk history will have a clear context.

Equally, if the person denies any ideas or plans about risk behaviours, there is more likely to be some evidence in the history for you to cite any concerns you have. For example, if the person has symptoms of clinical depression, describing difficulty in solving interpersonal problems, feeling trapped and seeing no hope for the future, yet then denies having even thought about suicide, the evidence base about depression and suicidal ideation would lead you to want to explore this more assertively as that would be unlikely, given those experiences.

Finally, having completed the assessment (as already detailed), you can then make a risk formulation and begin negotiating a risk management plan (Harrison and Hart, 2006).

Self rating

Asking the person to rate how they feel, whether this be about their mood or another element of their clinical presentation, can be useful in getting an immediate sense of its severity. For example, considering thoughts about harming someone else can open up more detail about the risk, as well as allowing an insight into the decision making process behind it (see clinical example 21).

Self rating can also be used to plot movement, or change. For example, when assessing someone's mood, you might begin by asking then to rate their mood on a scale of 1–10, with 10 being them feeling as well as they possibly could, and 1 being as low in mood as possible. If they tell you it's currently 4, you can check out the number that reflects their mood most of the time. That might be 7. You can see, therefore, how much of a change there has been from their normal mood. You can also check out what might need to happen if their mood were to improve to 5. Or, alternatively, what might cause it to drop to 3.

This can be married to ideas of self-harm. Do they recognise a number on their mood scale when they start to have ideas about self-harm or even suicide? Is there a number when they act upon those ideas?

Potential risk

The identification of future risk is not an easy task and will be open to interpretation, even between the person being assessed and the assessor. Thus the patient may have a particular perspective about the risks they face, some of which is shared by the assessor. However, you may have taken the view that the level of risk is either greater than the person thinks or that there are elements of their potential behaviour that poses risks with which they do not agree (see Figure 3.2., Johari's Window, below).

Johari's Window (1955) postulates that there are:

1. aspects of our personality known only to us, as individuals;
2. some we share with others;
3. some about which we have no insight but which are known to others;
4. others still that are still entirely unknown to the person and those around them.

Adapting this model to think about risk, the assessor faces some obvious challenges from the outset. Even if the person being assessed is forthcoming, there are likely to be some elements of risk about which the person will have limited or no understanding. While it may be relatively straightforward to discuss those aspects of risk that the patient can recognise, discussing the elements currently unknown will inevitably be difficult.

It may be someone understands the seriousness of their ideas to harm themselves but has no insight into behaviours that precipitate the risk or place them at risk in other ways. For example, a woman drinking and using illicit substances may not see how that leaves her sexually vulnerable and can increase the likelihood of her acting on suicidal thoughts. A person with psychotic phenomena may not link increased illicit substance misuse with an increase in their paranoia and subsequent violence.

Equally, the element of 'unknown to self and others' can act as a useful reminder that, even if you have addressed the risks previously unknown to the person, there may still be risk behaviours, or responses to situations, that neither the assessor or person being assessed have access to, which is what ultimately makes it so difficult to predict. This can only be addressed by asking the 'What if…?' question (see below).

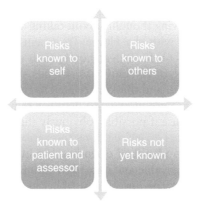

Figure 3.2 Johari's Window adapted for risk

'What if...?' scenario planning

The 'What if...?' question relates to scenario planning. Essentially, it is enquiring about:

- whether or not the person has, or is likely to develop, a 'plan "B"' if they cannot carry out their original plan;
- what will happen if anything changes;
- scenarios that could occur in certain circumstances;
- any unforeseen risks that have not occurred to the person being interviewed but might emerge if potential scenarios are put to them.

Inevitably, it might seem there is a degree of trying to make 'predictions' here but a lot of scenario planning will come from having gained knowledge about what has happened in the person's past, particularly exploring the detail of known risk factors and past patterns of risk behaviours, then looking at their current circumstances and how potential change(s) might affect future risk. This aids thinking about that area where risks are currently unknown to patient and assessor, and involves reasoned clinical judgement (Maden, 2007; Webster et al., 1997). Below are some scenarios to illustrate this.

Scenario 1: If... William is cutting his arms because he is ruminating about his situation and feels very tense and distressed, and an intervention is put in place to stop him doing this, how will he react? The act of stopping him from self-harming might actually lead to an increase in his ruminations and distress unless a healthier, more adaptive coping mechanism is provided to help him cope. In that situation, he may experience an increase in suicidal thoughts.

If he required admission to hospital, a different environment may help him feel calmer and more in control. But what if it doesn't and he not only remains preoccupied, tense and distressed but there is nothing in place to help him cope with this, until he feels completely overwhelmed? Is there a risk he may now try and kill himself by, for example, using something as a ligature as he has no access to tablets?

Scenario 2: If... Oliver is detained under the Mental Health Act on a forensic ward because he believes his thoughts are rational, his violence justified and that he doesn't need to take treatment, how will he react? Might he try and abscond? Might he pose a risk to staff if he wants to leave and believes they are unreasonably stopping him from doing so? How might an increase in his stress levels and reaction to feeling he's being treated unfairly affect him? Could he now also pose a risk to himself if his mood changes?

Scenario 3: What if... Emma doesn't want to be admitted onto an acute psychiatric ward as she says no one will do anything helpful for her there and that makes her feel worse? Although she is still having thoughts about taking an overdose of tablets at home, she says she will collaborate with the Home Treatment Team and remain safe.What might make things more difficult for her at home, such as another argument with her mother, a phone call from one of the university friends she thinks 'abandoned' her, an unpredicted change in her mood and thinking related to ruminations about past trauma? What might help? What things are in place to help her remain safe, e.g. removing dangerous medicines from the house if possible (obviously this doesn't remove all risk from the house but is both symbolic, i.e., we're taking this seriously, and practically addresses the one specific means she has identified of ending her life); seeking the support of her mother if that is practical, achievable and agreed by Emma; visits from the Home Treatment Team; access to a crisis or help line; the use of her local Emergency Department and mental health liaison team as a last resort. There needs to be an awareness of Emma's current risk and the plan to address this being clearly understood by all involved.

Key to this type of "What if...?" or scenario planning is that the team, having considered potential risks, now has to incorporate something into the risk management plan to try and prevent it happening. Suddenly the problem is not that the person *was* suicidal. They *are* suicidal and interventions have to be in place to address this. It is not that the person *was* violent in the community as a result of a psychotic breakdown but has been admitted into hospital and behaved safely throughout their time there. Will they be able to behave safely when discharged back into the community, and what might, specifically, increase the risk of violence? (see Part 5, Managing risk).

Considering potential risks involves exploring an adapted form of the issues listed in section two of Part 1 in the *Pocket Guide*, which are:

Early warning signs

How might we know the situation is building towards the person acting in a dangerous way?

Theoretically, this is easier with known patients. There should be a relapse profile, e.g. a chronology of events that previously led to a set of risk behaviours and risk event or near miss. On this point, it is just as important to note and learn from good practice, when a patient and team have avoided a serious incident, e.g. suicide attempt or act of violence, by proactively addressing the risk.

Nonetheless, potential risk has to be considered with newly referred and previously unknown patients. This is inevitably more speculative and difficult, especially with adolescents or people misusing substances because of the increased impulsivity, but still essential.

Key clinical tip

Because it hasn't yet happened, doesn't mean it won't. Always consider potential risks, what may make them more likely to be enacted and what might make it less likely the person will act.

What is the person likely to do?

If this is a violent act to others, what, specifically, would it be likely to be and is there anyone specific at risk? If the risk is to self, might it be self-harm or suicide? Might more than one person be at risk?

Motivation

It is important to understand the person's motivation for what they did or are thinking of doing, as well as how motivated they are to work with you in remaining safe. This means considering, with them:

- What was the problem (or, possibly, need) the person wants to address by self-harming or ending their life (as opposed to the problem clinicians and/or others are seeking to resolve)?

- Do they still see self-harm or suicide as the only means of doing this?
- If so, how strongly motivated are they to do that?
- If no longer wanting to self-harm or end their life, what does the person want to achieve now?
- How engaged are they in working with you to remain safe?
- Does your risk management plan correlate with the person's level of collaboration? (See Figure 3.3 below.)

If the problem the person is grappling with is that they find life unbearable and we are concerned with finding them accommodation, there is an obvious discrepancy. If we want the person to maintain their safety but they want to be dead, that has to be figured into our plan, as we certainly can't rely on that person to do 'what we want'.

Intent

What does the person think they will achieve – remembering the actual act might not achieve what the person intends. For example, someone may take an overdose of an anti-depressant believing it will be lethal. Unknown to them, it will not cause any significant medical effects but this does not negate the fact they wanted to die when they took the tablets. A person who thinks taking 20 Paracetamol tablets as a means of shutting out their psychic pain may not want to die but find the tablets prove lethal.

Severity

What would the likely consequences of the act be? Could it be life threatening? Would it have little significance?

Immediacy

Is the person likely to act as soon as they have an opportunity? If they are not immediately at risk, would certain things have to happen to change that?

Frequency

Is this something that would be limited to a 'one off' act? If the person were thwarted, would they try again? How quickly? If self-harm or violence, is it likely to be repetitive? Has a pattern already been established and, if so, is that understood by the person and others, e.g. clinicians working with them?

Duration

Are these risk behaviours likely to be present for a long time or related to specific events and, therefore, time limited? If related to specific events, are they likely to re-cur if something similar happens? Equally, if the stressors are of a chronic nature, e.g. poor interpersonal relationships, and therefore likely to create a constantly volatile environment which the person finds challenging, how will they maintain their safety within it?

Likelihood

Ultimately, perhaps the most difficult question is: how likely is it these risk behaviours will actually happen?

Considering how to manage actual and potential risks is detailed in Part 4 but needs to incorporate a range of issues (see Table 3.5).

Table 3.5 Questions to address potential risk and assist in scenario planning

---

1. What might make it more likely the person will act?
2. What might make it less likely the person will act?
3. How would you, as a clinician, know, i.e. what is your contact and relationship with the person?
4. Has something happened that means you need to re-assess the risk? (see Box 9).
5. What treatment(s) and specific interventions are in place to address and reduce the potential risk behaviours identified?
6. If there are specific individuals at risk, as well as the patient, what is needed to protect them?
7. Are you going to act now or do you need to act if certain circumstances change? (This brings you back to point 4.)
8. How frequently do you, with the clinical team, need to review the situation (as opposed to a re-assessment of the patient)?
9. How concerned are you about this person and does this case sit within your overall clinical priorities in terms of you putting sufficient resource and time into safely managing it?
10. Finally, is the person currently in the right environment for you to safety manage the potential risk behaviours with them?

Key clinical tip

Think about gaps in your knowledge about, and understanding of, the patient and potential risks. Why is something unclear? Is the patient withholding something, is it unclear to them, have you not asked the right questions or explored things in sufficient depth? Crucially, think of a strategy that will enable you to get the information you need or what you will do in its absence.

Specifics in assessing risk to self

The first thing to consider when assessing the risk an individual poses to themselves is whether it is suicide or self-harm. As noted in Part 2, these are very different, although there is a relationship between self-harm and suicide and the former can and does escalate to the latter, with most people who end their lives having self-harmed previously.

Key clinical tip

It is important to remember suicide and self-harm are not the same thing – self-harm can be used as a means to deflect suicidal ideation but people who self-harm can go on to kill themselves either accidentally or intentionally.

The act itself

We have explored above numerous ways in which potential risk can be explored. In cases where the person has self-harmed there are things we need to know at the end of the assessment to assist on our risk formulation and risk management plan (see Table 3.6 below).

A core part of the assessment of self-harm and/or suicide is linking the person's thoughts and emotions to the risk behaviour. Their importance is highlighted in Joiner's Model of Suicide and models such as Cry of Pain and Emotional Cascade (see Part 2, page 19). Exploring the sequence of events, e.g. Emma not getting messages from her friends about a planned night out, another argument with her mother and then walking over the bridge from which she would jump in the river, only tells a small part of her story. Her thoughts about her friends and their reasons for apparently 'abandoning' her, her thoughts about her mother and the reasons they argued, coupled with ruminating about disturbing memories and her overall cognitive schema (a framework or concept by which we organise and interpret information), are essential to understanding her as a person in a situation she was struggling to control. How those thoughts interacted with her emotions can help us understand her behaviour and interview techniques to help in that process are explored in clinical example 18.

The chronology and interaction of the person's thoughts and feelings are crucial to understanding their behaviour, as is a chronology of external events and their impact on the person's thoughts and feelings.

At the conclusion of the conversation, the clinician undertaking the assessment should have discovered the answer to the questions in Table 3.5, as well as those required to develop a risk formulation (see Part 4, Developing a risk formulation for more detail).

Table 3.6 25 essential things to find out from the assessment of self-harm and/or suicide

1. Why act now?
2. What events led to the act?
3. What protective factors had prevented it until now?
4. What changed?
5. Were there specific mental health related issues, e.g. depression, command hallucinations?
6. Was the person influenced by anyone else's actions?
7. Was it premeditated or impulsive?
8. If impulsive, what was the trigger?
9. If premeditated, how much planning was involved?
10. Did the person provide any 'warnings' beforehand?
11. Did they make any attempts to conceal their preparation?
12. What stopped the attempt, e.g. did the person stop of their own volition or due to external causes?
13. Were the means used, e.g. tablets, acquired for this specific attempt?
14. What was the person's intention, e.g. to die, escape from an intolerable situation?
15. What did the person think might happen as a consequence of their attempt?
16. How did the person think other people might have responded?
17. Was the attempt itself controlled or was there a loss of control?
18. What did the person do after the attempt, e.g. was there any attempt to tell anyone or seek help or were they found?
19. Did they try and conceal what they had done or deny it?
20. Have they been consistent in their account since being found to have self-harmed/attempted suicide?
21. Is there any way in which they are trying to minimise their actions?

22. How does the person feel now they have survived – do they regret what they did or are they unhappy to have survived?
23. If unhappy at surviving, are they acknowledging they would make a further attempt?
24. Do they now want help?
25. How collaborative are they likely to be?

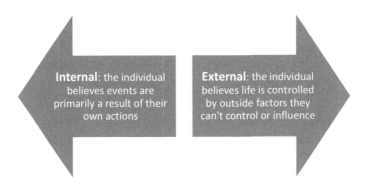

Figure 3.3 The locus of control

Locus of control

Locus of Control refers to an individual's perception about the underlying main causes of events in (their) life, though Julian Rotter (1966), who developed the concept, originally called it The Locus of Control and Reinforcement, as he thought behaviour was largely guided by reinforcements in the shape of rewards and punishments. Through these reinforcements, individuals develop beliefs about what causes their actions, which then influence the attitudes and behaviours the individual embraces. It runs as a continuum between an external locus of control to an internal locus of control (see Figure 3.3).

There are specific tools for assessing and measuring the locus of control. However, trying to understand how the person perceives they are affected by factors outside their control and which have contributed to their suicidal thinking or self-harm, or thinks they can influence things even at a difficult point in their life, will help you gain a better sense of risk and how that can be safely managed. Research suggests 'a clear association between locus of control and suicidal behaviour, with the individuals who had engaged in suicidal behaviours characterised by a more external locus of control' (Pearce and Martin, 1993). Examples below look at how someone's perception of their locus of control can be understood through the way they explain their rationale for their respective attempts to end their life.

Internal locus of control

William identifies his suicidal thoughts and actions are a consequence of his inability to bear his feelings, e.g. of loneliness, rejection, loss since Kelly left. He is thus identifying an internal cause for his behaviour. In conversation with the clinician, despite his current difficulties, he is able to come up with suggestions to help himself remain safe. The clinician can explore William's existing psychological and emotional coping mechanisms or previous ways in which he has coped with such difficult experiences and feelings, aiming to build upon these.

External locus of control

Emma perceives she has no choice other than to self-harm or attempt to end her life in reaction to the struggles in her relationship with her mother and apparent rejection by her university friends. She sees her behaviour as a direct consequence of what they have done and how it affects her. Since the clinician cannot get Emma's university friends to go out with her, or do anything at that time to change Emma's mother's behaviour in the way Emma may want it to change, the risk management plan has to take account of Emma's perception of her situation. Nor can the clinician rely on tapping into Emma's coping mechanisms as she sees her problems – and locus of control – as being external to her. This will increase the risk of further acts of self-harm and/or suicide attempts.

Psychosis

There is another element to consider when thinking about why the person may be at risk, and that is the impact of the person's mental disorder. This inevitably changes the person's thinking, feelings and perception of what is happening around them.

In clinical examples 19 and 21 (below) we will see comments by Oliver that strongly suggest he has an external locus of control, e.g. suggesting his violence is a consequence of others' actions, that 'it's their fault', they've 'got it coming' because of what they're doing'. Layered onto that are his incorrect and delusional beliefs that he is being 'infected' by others, that they are a threat to his safety.

This has led to Oliver assaulting Daniel and having thoughts about assaulting nursing staff as a result of delusional beliefs and auditory hallucinations that have worsened as he has become increasingly stressed. The clinician has to immediately address the psychosis as well as Oliver's cognitive and emotional response to what he perceives is happening.

Command hallucinations

It would be even more serious if Oliver were experiencing command hallucinations. Key questions then would include:

- When did he begin experiencing command hallucinations? (Remembering you would want to use non jargonistic language to do this, so might refer to it as 'voices, or a voice, that tell you what to do'.)
- How frequently does he experience hearing them?
- How does he feel about the experience? Does it frighten him? Does he want it to stop?
- Are there times they are worse or better? This could be at particular times of the day, or occasions, e.g. when particularly stressed.
- Is anything significant happening around him at the time?
- Who is talking to him? Is it a voice or voices he recognises? Does this ever change?
- Does he hear a variety of commands?
- What is their content, i.e. what does he actually hear the voices telling him? Does this change?
- Is he being told to do things he doesn't want to do? Is he being told to do anything dangerous?
- How intrusive are they? Can he distract himself from them?
- Is he able to resist some commands and not others?
- What is he able to do to stop himself acting upon the commands?

- Does he always act upon the commands he receives?
- If not always, what is different about those that he does follow and those he doesn't?
- Would he act upon instructions or commands that would be dangerous to himself and/ or others?

NB: it may be a patient reports acting upon command hallucinations but that these are currently relatively safe. It is crucial to explore what might happen if the commands became more dangerous and plan for such a contingency. There will also be a wide range of factors beyond Oliver's control, such as external stressors that may exacerbate the auditory hallucinations. The risks here are extremely serious.[i] There is some evidence that the more authoritative the person articulating the commands is, the more likely the person receiving them is to act upon them.

A recognised assessment tool for exploring psychosis, useful for an in depth assessment, may not be practical when conducting a risk assessment. Its absence should not delay the risk assessment or assessment of the person's psychotic phenomena.

Other questions to explore when considering why the person is at risk include:

- Is there a pattern?
- Is there a risk profile?
- Do certain events or responses exacerbate or improve the situation?
- What are the warning signs? Does the person know when things are getting worse and when they are more at risk? How would others, including those caring for them, know?

Another aspect of the assessment to consider includes less obvious factors that will impact upon many people who self-harm or act dangerously. These include:

- poor negotiating skills;
- difficulties in problem solving, particularly in the context of interpersonal relationships;
- susceptibility to stress;
- lack of assertiveness;
- lack of social skills;
- peer influence.

The prevalence and severity of these factors needs to be taken into account when thinking about risk management (McGranaghan, 2004). For example, how successful is a risk management plan likely to be if it relies on the patient solving quite complex or challenging problems?

Impulsivity

Suicide rarely, if ever, occurs without the person having thought about it, how they might do it and some degree of planning, even if this is limited to someone considering a ligature thinking about whether or not they have a rope, what they might attach it to and how they would tie the knot. However, some people who survive a suicide attempt will describe the final decision to act as an impulsive phenomenon, a sudden response to a particular trigger that sets in motion the taking of tablets or cutting or going to a physical place to end their life (see, for example, www.kevin.hines.com).

This impulse can be transient. If support is available close to or at the moment of impulse, there is the possibility the crisis may be defused, as is discussed in Part 2.

Assessing how impulsive someone is likely to be is, therefore, essential, particularly as while they may act 'on impulse' after an apparently innocuous event or trigger, the person usually has at least the basis of a plan in place that could be lethal. Of course, drugs and/ or alcohol may play a part in this as they decrease inhibition and increase impulsivity. The heightened impulsivity of adolescents also has to be factored in, discussed and, when there is no history of self-harm or suicide, explored through other situations, relationships or parts of their life that might give an indication of their potential for sudden risk behaviours.

Another element to impulsivity is the risk of 'opportunistic' self-harm. The person may act upon ideas already formed but not into a developed plan because the opportunity presents itself at time of high arousal.

Rigidity

When feeling suicidal, people are usually constricted in their thinking, mood and action. Their reasoning is dichotomised and, in exploring possible alternatives to death with the suicidal patient, the clinician has to aim to help the person realise there are other options, even if they don't seem ideal to that person at the time.

Assessing the risk to others

While the principles of assessing risk to others are the same as exploring any other domain of risk, there can be differences in the process and context of the discussion and dynamic between assessor and person being assessed. Unlike the exploration of most other areas of risk assessment, there are possible implications for the criminal justice system (and Mental Health Act) when discussing dangerousness to others, whether potential or actual. The person you're interviewing is almost certainly going to be aware of this, potentially making self disclosure harder and how you approach it, as the assessor, potentially more complicated. Nonetheless, the assessor should still aim to find out as much as possible about the risk as in any other assessment (see Table 3.6).

Table 3.7 25 essential things to find out from the assessment of violence

---

1. Why act now?
2. What led up to the incident?
3. What protective factors had prevented it until now?
4. What changed?
5. Were there specific mental health related issues, e.g. depression, command hallucinations?
6. Was the person the main perpetrator or did they become involved due to the influence of another?
7. Did they encourage anyone else's participation?
8. Was it premeditated or impulsive?
9. If it was premeditated, how much planning was involved?
10. If impulsive, what was the trigger?
11. Were there threats beforehand?
12. Did they make any attempts to conceal their preparation?
13. What stopped the violence, e.g. did the person stop of their own volition or due to external causes, such as being restrained?
14. If a weapon was used, was it habitually carried or used for that specific assault?

15. What was the person's intention when carrying out the assault?
16. Was the violence controlled or was there a loss of control?
17. Was there any element of sadism, e.g. was there any element of torture or attempt to dominate?
18. What did the person do afterwards?
19. Did they try and conceal their involvement, admit to the violence or deny it?
20. How were they caught?
21. Have they been consistent in their account since being found to have been violent?
22. Is there any way in which they are trying to minimise their actions?
23. To whom/what does the person attribute responsibility, e.g. the victim, co-perpetrators, circumstances etc?
24. What is the person's attitude towards the violence now?
25. How collaborative are they likely to be?

As with other areas of the person's biographical story, and risk assessment, start with historical details – this is not just asking if the patient has been in trouble with the police or has convictions, but:

• Have they done anything that might have resulted in police action had the police known about it?
• If so, what did they do and in what context?
• Have they been involved in acts of violence in the past?
• Again, what was the context?
• Have they used weapons?
• Do they routinely carry weapons?

See also: 'The act itself' (page 152), which looks at the level of detail that needs to be explored in the light of an assault on someone else.

Clinical example 19 looks at how to progress a conversation with Oliver after he has assaulted a fellow patient.

Clinical Example 19:   Addressing risk to others

Clinician: Thanks for that. I want to move on, if that's okay?
Oliver: If you want.
Clinician: You mentioned that you got in some trouble when you were at school. Did that involve the police?
Oliver: What, like being arrested?
Clinician: Yes.
Oliver: No.
Clinician: Was it the sort of thing – or has there been anything else – that might have got you in trouble with the police if it had come to their attention?
Oliver: [*Pause*] I'm not sure what you mean.
Clinician: Maybe getting into fights or doing anything illegal.
Oliver: [*Pause*] I did a bit of shoplifting when I was a kid.

Clinician:	What sort of things?
Oliver:	Just stuff. Nothing much.
Clinician:	Was it for you or stuff you could sell?
Oliver:	Bit of both.
Clinician:	How did you get into that?
Oliver:	An older kid used to do it. I used to hang out with him. He showed me how to do it.
Clinician:	Did you always do it together?
Oliver:	No. He used to keep everything for himself so I went off on my own.
Clinician:	You were saying earlier that you've used a lot of cannabis and cocaine in the past but hadn't been able to find work. Did you ever have to steal things so you could buy drugs?
Oliver:	A bit. Everyone does that.
Clinician:	Did you ever sell drugs so you could buy your own?
Oliver:	I can't remember. Anyway, I cut right down. I knew it was getting out of hand.
Clinician:	Were there any other things?
Oliver:	Things?
Clinician:	Things you did that might have got you into trouble…
Oliver:	Ah. One or two arguments. Nothing serious.
Clinician:	Did they ever become physical?
Oliver:	Not really. I only defend myself. If I'm being threatened, you know?
Clinician:	What happened?
Oliver:	This guy was going to do things to me.
Clinician:	How did you know that? Was it something he said?
Oliver:	He didn't have to.
Clinician:	But you knew?
Oliver:	Oh yeah. The way he was looking, the way he was standing.
Clinician:	What did you think he was going to do?
Oliver:	Mess up my head. Infect me.
Clinician:	How was he going to do that?
Oliver:	Put stuff in me. I don't know.
Clinician:	What did you do?
Oliver:	Hit him. He had it coming. Shouldn't have done that.
Clinician:	Did you punch him or use a weapon?
Oliver:	I punched him a couple of times… He'd been enjoying himself, getting at me. So maybe I punched him when he went down. But I ran off before anyone could grab me.
Clinician:	Is that what led to you coming into hospital?
Oliver:	No. I was stitched up by my CPN. He told the psychiatrist and social worker stuff about me that wasn't true.
Clinician:	So, there have been incidents when you've felt you needed to defend yourself and that led to you hitting people. [*Pause*] Are there times you've used a weapon?

Oliver:	Like I said, only to defend myself.
Clinician:	What did you use?
Oliver:	I used a strap wrapped around my fist. It makes it more painful when you hit them and you don't hurt your hand as much. I hit someone with a bottle once but it didn't break. In fact I hit him twice. [*Laughs*] He had a right hard head. I got a good kicking for that.
Clinician:	When was that?
Oliver:	About five years ago. I haven't done anything like that since. [*Pause*] Well...
Clinician:	There was something else?
Oliver:	Yeah. Sort of.
Clinician:	What happened on that occasion?
Oliver:	it wasn't much. Some guy was having a go at this dancer in a club. He was shouting out about her being ugly. That was out of order.
Clinician:	What did you do?
Oliver:	I glassed him.
Clinician:	What do you mean?
Oliver:	You know. I smashed a glass in his face.
Clinician:	Was he badly hurt?
Oliver:	Dunno. I didn't hang around to find out. There was some blood. Who knows?
Clinician:	Anything else?
Oliver:	A guy in a pub. He was jealous. Of what I've done, what I've got. His girlfriend was staring at me. She could see what I was thinking, you know, about what I wanted to do to her. She loved it. He didn't. I knew what was coming so I hit him first.
Clinician:	Have you ever carried a weapon?
Oliver:	[*Pause*] Sometimes.
Clinician:	What was happening that you did that?
Oliver:	In case someone was after me.
Clinician:	Was that a concern about anyone in particular?
Oliver:	No. It could have been anyone. You never know, do you? You got to protect yourself.
Clinician:	What did you carry with you?
Oliver:	It was only one of those jacknife things. You know, one you can open up. I never had to use it.
Clinician:	Do you think you would have used it?
Oliver:	If I had to. 'Course. You know, If someone's doing stuff to me, messing up my head. I wouldn't have used it against someone like that clown in the pub.
Clinician:	Why did you stop carrying it?
Oliver:	I nearly got stopped by the police a couple of times so I threw it in the river. I didn't want to get nicked.
Clinician:	How did you manage to feel safe without it?

Oliver:	I didn't. I was always on edge. I had to be really careful about where I went and who was about.
Clinician:	Is that when you started using cannabis a bit more?
Oliver:	Yeah. It helps. Takes the edge off things. Chills me.

In this lengthy example, the clinician simply follows the story without commenting on the behaviours or indicating any personal views about it, which enables him to gather more information. From this, the clinician now has a clear understanding of the motivating factors for Oliver's violence and a number of risks are elicited:

1. Oliver has a history of violent assaults on strangers in response to psychotic phenomena but will also get into arguments and use violence when not psychotic.
2. He has routinely carried a weapon to protect himself and would have used it.
3. He has been involved in theft and the buying and selling of drugs.
4. He minimises his violence and other dangerous behaviours and doesn't readily volunteer information.
5. He displays no remorse for his violence.
6. He derives at least a degree of gratification and pleasure from his violence.

All of these factors, and the information gleaned in clinical examples 19, 20 and 21, can feature in the assessment of risk and its management.

As noted above, asking the use of self rating can be helpful both in detailing the level of risk as well as opening out the discussion about the nature of the risk, the likelihood of the person acting upon their ideas and the context in which that might happen (see clinical example 20).

Clinical Example 20:   Using a rating scale

Clinician:	You were telling me that you had been thinking about hitting Daniel for a few days.
Oliver:	Yeah.
Clinician:	You were thinking about it but didn't feel like you had to do anything at that time?
Oliver:	No.
Clinician:	What changed?
Oliver:	Right. He'd been staring at me. Like, trying to get at me. Like, 'I can eat your soul'. You know? That kind of crap. Then, he changes his mind–
Clinician:	How could you tell?
Oliver:	It was obvious. I could feel it. He started trying to infect me. That's when we had the argument... it's hard to explain... but after that I couldn't get the idea out of my head...
Clinician:	I wonder if we can use a scale to help us work out the difference. Can you tell me how strong the thoughts were, on a scale of

	1–10, with 1 being not strong at all and 10 meaning they couldn't have been any stronger? So, before the argument, how strong were they?
Oliver:	Well, I really didn't want to hit him. I mean, I did. I'd think about it, if I saw him, like. But I wasn't that bothered.
Clinician:	You threatened him.
Oliver:	That was just to wind him up. So… maybe a 6.
Clinician:	Then things changed.
Oliver:	When he's decided he's going to infect me and take control of me. That makes everything different. Like I said, I couldn't stop thinking about it, even though I knew I shouldn't and… well, I still didn't really want to…
Clinician:	What number would you put to it?
Oliver:	8. Maybe 9.
Clinician:	That's a big jump. And that was why you went on to hit him?
Oliver:	Yeah. Of course.
Clinician:	At what number do you think the thoughts become so strong, that you're not going to be able to stop yourself from acting on them?
Oliver:	Um, I'm not sure. Maybe 7.
Clinician:	So it sounds as if you carried on resisting for quite a while?
Oliver:	Yeah.
Clinician:	Why was that?
Oliver:	I knew I'd get into trouble.
Clinician:	Oliver, this has really been useful in helping me understand what happens. I've just got a couple more questions.
Oliver:	Go on then.
Clinician:	Once you get to 7, you're not going to be able to stop yourself?
Oliver:	No. it's right inside my head by then. And I'm, I don't know, all those things are happening to my body. I have to stop them happening.
Clinician:	And what number are you at most of the time?
Oliver:	[*Pause*] I don't know. That's a good question. Er, I guess I go between a 4 and a 5. Mostly 5.
Clinician:	It doesn't take a lot to move you up to that point of no return then? You don't have a lot of space…
Oliver:	No. It's like I'm full up most of the time. Full. That's the only way I can explain it.
Clinician:	Why do you think you're at 5 most of the time? That's high.
Oliver:	Is it? Yeah. Well, there's… I'm not sure. You have to be able to protect yourself, don't you? if you relax… anything can happen. There's people just waiting for me to drop my guard, to take advantage. I can't take any chances.
Clinician:	And it feels like that most of the time?
Oliver:	Yeah.
Clinician:	Maybe that's what we can work at – helping you feel less 'full'.

This conversation allows the clinician to gain an insight into Oliver's usual state of readiness to be violent, when his thoughts about it become more intense and the number at which he can't stop himself from acting upon his thoughts, before reaching the point at which he will actually be violent. This can figure into the risk management plan and possibly also help Oliver communicate his state of readiness to be violent. Other things emerge. It certainly appears from this conversation that one of the factors in his change in thinking about acting violently is his perception that Daniel now presents as an active threat to him, i.e. '...going to infect me and take control of me'. It's also clear that, much of the time, he is feeling that he has to be 'on his guard', ready to protect himself and with the potential for violence, apparently linked to his mental state.

Clinical Example 21:   Exploring attitudes to violence

Clinician: Thinking about the people you hit–
Oliver: It wasn't like I did it for nothing. It wasn't down to me. Besides, it's not a big deal. I hope you're not going to use this against me.
Clinician: Well, I need to share it with the team. But I did explain that at the beginning. I was wondering how you felt after you'd hit those people.
Oliver: All right. How am I supposed to feel? They deserved it. I told you that. I was only defending myself.
Clinician: Did you enjoy it in any way?
Oliver: [*Pause*] A bit, I suppose, now you ask. I never really thought that much about it. Not always.
Clinician: Do you know if any of them were badly hurt?
Oliver: No. Well, I don't know. I told you about the guy I glassed. The bloke I hit with the bottle, even though the bottle didn't break, his head was still cut up. But his mates did me over for that, didn't they? And Dan, you make out like it's a big deal. He was asking for it, don't you get that? And yeah, there was a bit of blood. Good. I'm glad. You want to know the truth? I wish I'd shanked him for what he was trying to do.

Clinical example 21 highlights Oliver's lack of remorse about his violence, the way he minimises both his actions and their impact as well as his sense of justification, and a means of defending himself. This all suggests the risk of violence remains both immediate and serious and that a risk management plan is likely to require a degree of imposition, certainly in terms of needing to treat his psychosis, as this is inextricably linked to his current violence.

If you suspect the person poses a risk to others, it is important to be as specific as possible and use interviewing techniques aimed at opening up the conversation. Clinical example 22 shows some of the potential problems in using certain types of question.

Clinical Example 22:   Probing ongoing risk to others

Closed questions:

Clinician:	Are you thinking about harming anyone on the ward?
Oliver:	No.

Leading questions:

Clinician:	Why do you want to hurt Daniel?
Oliver:	I never said I was going to do that.

Open questions and funnelling in:

Clinician:	How have you been today, Oliver?
Oliver:	All right.
Clinician:	Has that been all day?
Oliver:	I dunno. Most of it. Why?
Clinician:	I noticed you and Daniel had what looked like a difficult conversation.
Oliver:	Did it?
Clinician:	Was it? A difficult conversation, I mean?
Oliver:	Not really.
Clinician:	I might have been wrong but I thought you looked quite upset at the time, and afterwards you went back to your room and were playing your music loudly and pacing around.
Oliver:	So?
Clinician:	I know, in the past, you've said you play your music loudly if you're not feeling great. I wondered if that was anything to do with the conversation with Daniel.
Oliver:	Well, he's a pain, you know?
Clinician:	I'm not sure. Can you tell me about that?
Oliver:	Like this morning, I just asked him for something, you know, something simple, and he starts ranting and raving, just dissing me for no reason.
Clinician:	How did you feel when he was doing that?
Oliver:	I was angry. You would have been. He's at it.
Clinician:	What?
Oliver:	Messing with my head. [*Pause*] Look. If someone is going to hurt me, I'm going to have to defend myself. Right?
Clinician:	Is that what you were thinking this morning?
Oliver:	Maybe.
Clinician:	Is it because you feel more stressed?
Oliver:	Of course it is. It is stressful. Don't you know that?
Clinician:	Tell me more about it.

Oliver:	You know about how he stares at me, and he puts stuff inside me. Normally, he says he's not doing it, like he's some kind of saint.
Clinician:	Do you feel you need to do anything about that?
Oliver:	[*Long pause*] No.
Clinician:	You mentioned a while ago having thoughts about Daniel – and some of the nurses. I wondered if you still think about them.
Oliver:	Sometimes.
Clinician:	You think about harming Daniel?
Oliver:	Like I said, he's making threats to me, you know, what am I s'posed to do?
Clinician:	And which nurses do you think about?
Person:	Why do you want to know?
Clinician:	Because I'm worried about you and what might happen if you do try and harm someone [*pause*]. I'm worried about them. Can you tell me who it is?
Oliver:	You should know.
Clinician:	Why do you say that?
Oliver:	Because of what they're doing.
Clinician:	Would you tell me anyway?
Oliver:	Ola. And Jane.
Clinician:	Is there anyone else?
Oliver:	No.
Clinician:	Are you thinking about harming them now?
Oliver:	What? Right *now*? No.
Clinician:	But what about today or the last couple of days?
Oliver:	Yeah. See, Dan's gone into one and Jane is looking at me, smiling. And yesterday, she and Ola were talking about me. What right have they got to do that?
Clinician:	And this is about what you fear they might do to you?
Oliver:	Yeah, messing up my head and all that stuff. That's what they were talking about. With Dan. And I saw them laughing in the office. They write stuff down about me. In their computers. That goes up on the internet so everyone can read it and it's all lies.
Clinician:	Lots of us write things about you, Oliver.
Oliver:	You know what I mean. Not like them.
Clinician:	Hmm. That's helpful. How do you know which of us isn't writing bad stuff about you, or trying to infect you?
Oliver:	That's easy. The way people stand. The way they look at me, the expression on their face, talk. I just know.
Clinician:	You absolutely know?
Oliver:	Yeah. 'Course I do.
Clinician:	What about me, for instance?
Oliver:	You've always been all right. I've always liked you. Not like them and the things they do. It's vile.

Clinician:	What might you do about it?
Oliver:	I don't know.
Clinician:	What do you think about doing?
Oliver:	[*Pause*] I'd hit them, wouldn't I?
Clinician:	Would you use a weapon?
Oliver:	Might.
Clinician:	It might be hard to say, but do you think something might happen and you would 'snap', you know, do something without planning?
Oliver:	Yeah. I nearly did that this morning.
Clinician:	Have you thought about how you might try and hurt them though?
Oliver:	I'd only do it because I had to.
Clinician:	And what would you do?
Oliver:	I'd wait 'til they were on their own and maybe use hot water, out of the boiler. That would make them stop.
Clinician:	What would have to happen for you to do that?
Oliver:	Not much. I'm ready now. I don't care what happens to me anymore.

Here, through a slower pace, asking a variety of questions, the clinician keeps returning to the question of who is at risk and, particularly, what Oliver might do, as well as what might prompt him to act. Ultimately, she establishes he is likely to act on his thoughts through a very violent attack, even if that might be prompted by something that would make it appear more spontaneous. This would be far more difficult if after hitting a metaphorical brick wall by starting off with a closed question, which invites 'no' as an answer, and a leading question that is not based on anything that has yet been established.

Having used open questions to help Oliver open up, he goes on to give a clear picture of the effect of his delusional beliefs without ever being asked any direct questions about them. Simply by letting him talk about his beliefs the full extent of them emerges, as well as some of his reasoning, e.g. he is entitled to be violent to those trying to 'infect him', as well as how he decides who is a threat to him. Unlike in clinical example 11, when she had to rescue the situation after Oliver assumed she didn't believe him because of her choice of words, she is careful to ask about how he knows which of the staff *aren't* trying to do things to him, thus making it easier to explore this without the risk of alienating him and even feels confident enough to ask him how he feels about her, given the rapport they have established.

Given the psychotic nature of Oliver's presentation and the way in which he misinterprets others' actions, knowing exactly what someone may do that would prompt an attack is far more difficult.[ii] However, this does not mean an attack is unpredictable. In fact, we can conclude it is very likely to happen unless preventative action is taken. Given the biggest causal factor is Oliver's psychosis, and that this is most likely to increase when he is very stressed and/or psychologically aroused, actively treating that while at the same time minimising the amount of stress and stimulation he experiences must be a key part of the risk management plan.

At the same time, decisions have to be made about whether or not Oliver needs to be moved elsewhere. This invites a different – but equally serious – risk as he is likely to develop similar suspicions about others wherever he goes. At the same time, it may reinforce his paranoia and there is also a further risk of not knowing which people are the focus of his paranoia and potential violence. The other option is to move Daniel, Ola and Jane for their own protection.

It may be possible to keep them all on the ward together, with a very carefully worked out plan about which everyone was confident and willing to participate in. This would rely on having sufficient staff on duty, being able to know the whereabouts of all concerned at all times and the means to evaluate Oliver's safety on an ongoing basis while actively treating him. To assist in this decision, knowing why he hasn't been violent is useful (see clinical example 23).

Clinical Example 23:   Probing the build up to violence

Clinician: There are times you're not violent though.
Oliver: What do you mean?
Clinician: There must be times you're having these thoughts and feel unsafe, but you don't hit anyone.
Oliver: Yeah. 'Course. I want to get out of here. Look, I don't want aggravation, right?
Clinician: How do you stop yourself? You're having the thoughts, starting to move up the scale. What helps you avoid hitting someone?
Oliver: I do other stuff?
Clinician: What would you do?
Oliver: I dunno. I go back to my room. Play music with my headphones on. Someone taught me this thing, where you focus on what you can see, touch, hear. You know?
Clinician: Yes. Is there anything else that helps?

[*Oliver lists more coping mechanisms*]
Clinician: How would we know these weren't working for you?
Oliver: [*Smiles*] I'd hit someone.
Clinician: Before that?
Oliver: Um, I get irritable. Don't want to talk to people. I've been told I start staring at people. Then I start getting into arguments 'cause I've had enough of being dissed and treated like a mug. When thing are getting worse, I go back to my room but I know I pace about. I can't relax. I put my headphones on but I'll be talking to myself, like I've lost my mind. Sometime I bang my head on the wall, see if that might stop it all. Then I take my glasses off.
Clinician: Why do you do that?
Oliver: I don't want them to get broken in the fight when you lot come bundling in on me.

Now the clinician has a good idea of both coping strategies Oliver uses and warning signs that an assault on someone might be imminent. These can then be incorporated into a conversation about a risk management plan and, hopefully, the plan itself.

To summarise, in fully assessing risk to others, as much information as possible is required, including:

- what thoughts the person has about harming others;
- Who, if anyone specific, the person is thinking about harming;
- how they might harm the person, e.g. would they use a weapon and if so, what;
- in what circumstances might they harm the person;
- what might stop the person acting upon their thoughts.

If there has been violence:

- Why now?
- What were the events leading up to it?
- Were there specific mental health related issues?
- Were drugs and/or alcohol factors?
- Was the person the main perpetrator or did they become involved due to the influence of another person?
- Did they encourage anyone else's participation?
- Was the act premeditated or impulsive?
- If it was premeditated, how much planning was involved?
- If impulsive, what was the trigger?
- Were there threats beforehand?
- What stopped the violence, e.g. did the person stop of their own volition or due to external causes?
- Did the person have to be physically stopped from continuing the assault?
- If they hadn't been stopped, how much further might they have gone?
- What was their intention, e.g. using the minimum violence possible to prevent someone doing something and then stopping once that objective was achieved or, at the other end of the spectrum, to carry on until the other person was dead?
- If a weapon was used, was it habitually carried or used for that specific assault?
- Was the violence controlled or was there a loss of control?
- Was there any element of sadism, e.g. did they enjoy being violent and hurting their victim, was there any element of torture or attempt to dominate?

The biggest predictor of future violence is a history of violence, followed by intent, feasibility and capacity (or lack of it). In many cases where you are assessing someone's violence, it will be necessary to get a corroborating account given the likelihood that the person being assessed will minimise the event. Substance misuse and certain personality disorders as well as, to a much lesser extent, psychosis will also increase the likelihood of violence (Maden 2007, 2013).

After the violence:

- What did the person do afterwards?
- How were they discovered to have been violent? E.g. did their victim identify them, did they tell others about it?

- Did they attempt to cover up or conceal their violence?
- Did they admit to the violence or deny it?
- To whom/what does the person attribute responsibility? E.g. the victim, co-perpetrators, circumstances etc.?
- What is the person's attitude towards the violence now?
- Have they shown any remorse?

If someone specific is at risk:

- Does that person know?
- Who will notify them?
- Do the police need to be informed?
- It is also important to identify the nature of the violence the person is planning or contemplating. For example, have weapons been used or are they likely to be?
- If it emerges that the person has used/uses weapons, might they have one with them now and are you safe to continue the assessment?

Key clinical tip

Detail is absolutely crucial in assessing risk to others, as with all elements of risk assessment. The more information about the potential risk, the more robust the risk management plan can be.

Dealing with weapons

If someone has a weapon with him, you should follow your local policy on how to deal safely with this situation. If your team does not have one, that should be addressed as soon as possible (see Section Two above).

A safety first approach is *essential*. Unless you are extremely confident you can safely remove the weapon from the setting, you should remove yourself. However, even this is not without risk and simply 'running away', which might be your initial thought, is rarely an option unless you are directly confronted and have no other choice. In part, your decision will be guided by how physiologically aroused the person appears to be – but remember, someone who appears to be outwardly perfectly calm might still be preparing to attack. You may need to address it by direct questions, e.g.:

- "Do you have a weapon with you now?"
- "What do you have?"
- "Where is it?"

If it is in a bag or not on the person, e.g. somewhere in the room, you can ask if you can remove it. If you do so, you'll need to hand it to a colleague if in a hospital or clinic setting. If at home, you would need to know it was in another room that the person agrees they will not access (remembering that people's homes have numerous things that could be used as a weapon) but should terminate the interview and leave at the earliest possible moment. If there is any thought the person will use a weapon, or has one, the police should be informed as soon as possible.

Should the weapon be with the person and they want to give it to you, ask that it be placed in a neutral part of the room, e.g. on the table, and then take it from there. Do not allow the person to hand it to you directly.

If you suspect a person has a weapon but they either deny this or will not allow it to be removed, you should quietly but firmly terminate the interview and withdraw immediately, seeking assistance.

Key clinical tip

If you have any concerns about a person having a weapon before commencing an assessment – don't commence the assessment. Either have the weapon removed or involve the police immediately. If you begin to suspect the person has a weapon, address the issue and either remove the weapon if safe to do so or terminate the interview and seek assistance.

Brief assessments and re-assessments – the key principles

As stated earlier, one of the key principles to an effective risk assessment is devoting the necessary time to it. However, there will inevitably be occasions when the clinician has to make a brief assessment. Equally, a comprehensive assessment may have taken place in the recent past but there is now a need to re-assess without taking the patient through a repetitive and lengthy process. Other occasions that merit a brief exploration of risk are when this is a triage prior to recommending a fuller assessment from another healthcare professional, e.g. carried out by a member of an Emergency Department team prior to referral to a psychiatric liaison nurse.

The key components for a brief assessment are:

- The history of the presenting complaint, i.e. what has recently happened to prompt this presentation and why is it significant now?
- A summation of their current social situation and how it impacts on current risk, e.g.:
  - important relationships;
  - the type of accommodation they're living in and anyone they're living with;
  - employment or education;
  - social support;
  - any stressors, e.g. financial worries, bullying, recent loss.
- Relevant medical and psychiatric history.
- Current drug and alcohol use.
- Brief mental state examination, e.g. any obvious evidence of depression, anxiety, psychosis etc.
- Risk to self and/or others, both historical and current (to include information highlighted in the introduction. i.e. who, what, when, where, why and how), as well as:
  - immediacy;
  - severity;
  - intent;

- plan;
- level of collaboration;
- warning signs.

- Risk formulation.
- Risk management plan (Harrison and Hart, 2006).

The ACCEPT model

The ACCEPT model is a simple tool that can be used as a prompt for non mental health clinicians making observations of the person and possibly exploring elements of someone's mental state as part of a risk assessment or even triage. The acronym ACCEPT (see Table 3.8) stands for:

Appearance

Conduct

Communication

Emotions

Perceptions

Thoughts

Table 3.8 The ACCEPT model for brief mental health assessment (adapted from work by James Tighe)

Appearance
- How are they dressed?
- Grooming/hygiene
- Posture
- Facial expression
- Gait (how the person walks)
- Evidence of self-harm

Conduct (or behaviour)
- Eye contact
- Body language/gestures/movement
- Are they quiet and withdrawn?
- Arousal – is the person agitated or distressed?
- Ability to follow requests and instructions
- Rapport and engagement – do they volunteer information?

Communication
- Rate – is it fast or slow, difficult to interrupt or hard to get a response?
- Tone – is it monotonous, 'bouncy' etc?
- Volume – loud or soft
- Clarity – is what they're saying understandable, vague or incoherent?
- Quantity – saying a lot or very little?

Emotions
- Are they:
  - angry/irritable;
  - anxious;
  - 'low' or depressed;
  - elated;
  - apathetic;
  - labile – rapidly changing?

Perceptions
- How do they interpret what is happening around them?
- Are they hallucinating or having 'odd experiences'?
- Are their perceptions disturbing?
- **Do they feel safe?**

Thoughts
- Are their thoughts speeded up or slowed down?
- Are there unwanted, negative thoughts?
- Is there no logical sense?
- Is there a lot of irrelevant material?
- Does the person keep going off at a tangent?
- Is the person ruminating (thinking of the same thing, over and over)?
- Are they having violent thoughts/fantasies or thoughts about suicide and/or self-harm?

Not all of these questions and/or observations have to be part of a brief re-assessment or triage but can be used in order to give the clinician seeing the patient a structure and reference point for the process, as well as a guide to what they see and hear, along with any questions they decide to ask.

Triage

Triage refers to the assignment of degrees of urgency to wounds or illnesses to decide the order of treatment of patients. It is a key element of the structure of the overall service provided by staff in an Emergency Department but can also be used by different services, e.g. mental health emergency services. It is also similar to the process undertaken in a reception screening in a prison setting.

The task of the triage clinician is to go through a similar process they would with any other patient, i.e. to gather the maximum amount of information needed only to determine the patient's clinical pathway. The purpose is to gain an understanding of:

- Is the person fit for interview?
- Why are they presenting now?
- The specific nature of the risk(s).
- Their potential seriousness and immediacy.
- Is the person safe where they are?
- The level of their collaboration.
- Were they to want to discontinue the process and/or leave, do you think they will be safe to do so?
- Have they capacity?

Will a more in depth assessment be required? If that is the case, the triage clinician does not want the patient to have to repeat much of the information, hence not asking too many questions at this stage. To help the patient participate as fully as possible they should be told about:

- the purpose of this interview;
- the taking of basic observations, why this is happening and the results;
- why it will be brief;
- what will happen afterwards.

The triage clinician should then focus on elements of the key components detailed above without going into detail. It should not be expected that a non mental health clinician should be competent to assess someone's mental state nor even necessary but, given the number of people now presenting to Emergency Departments with mental health problems, it would clearly be useful for staff to receive sufficient education for them to be able to recognise the key symptoms of depression, anxiety and psychosis and feel confident to inform anyone coming in to do a full assessment of any concerns or issues picked up during the triage.

Re-assessments

Re-assessment should be seen as a routine part of the risk assessment and risk management cycle, particularly given the recognition of risk as a dynamic process. It is not just about the individual and their own mental, emotional and psychological state, attitudes and behaviour. The context and situation in which the individual is functioning needs constant attention and consideration, as these external factors can have a profound affect on risk (see Box 9). The crucial thing to explore is what has changed since the last assessment and whether or not this increases any previously identified risks or leads to consideration of new risk.

Box 9:   Occurrences that should prompt a re-assessment of risk

These would include:

- when a clinician or clinical team receive a referral of a person previously known to the service;
- when a person is transferred into a new team or service;
- briefly, before and after the patient has a period of leave;
- following a serious incident or an event that changes the context in which risk behaviours may occur;
- in anticipation of events that are known to increase risk, e.g. bereavement, significant change in relationships etc;
- before and after any significant change in treatment and/or the patient's management;
- at every Mental Health Act assessment and when considering discharging a patient from a section of the Act;
- prior to stepping down, e.g. from a psychiatric intensive care unit to acute inpatient unit, discharge from hospital to a community service and, for community services, upon working with a newly discharged patient.

Notes

i John Barrett was a patient under the care of a forensic team who perpetrated a homicide while experiencing command hallucinations. The case highlights the risks associated with this condition and requirements for thorough assessment of mental state and risk assessment. A full report of the tragedy can be found at: https://www.hundredfamilies.org/wp/wp-content/uploads/2021/05/JOHN-BARRETT-SEPT-04-lr.pdf.

ii There may, however, be some reality at the root of some of Oliver's ideas. He may have a very bad relationship with Daniel and Daniel may, indeed, be doing things which Oliver finds difficult, e.g. arguing with him, talking about him to other patients in a derogatory manner, trying to intimidate him etc., which is another reason to validate the feelings he has rather than how he interprets events and what he does in response to them. Equally, there may be issues about the body language of some of the nursing staff, how they stand with patients etc., their facial expression or even expressing negative attitudes towards Oliver that he has incorporated into his psychotic world. These obviously give his beliefs a basis in reality and would need to be addressed with the staff. While none of this can be used as an excuse or rationale for Oliver's violence, it can help understand how he arrived at the decisions he did and, therefore, what can be done to address this.

References and selected bibliography

Aldridge, D. (1997) *Suicide: The Tragedy of Hopelessness*, London: Jessica Kingsley.

Beck, A.T., Steer, R.A., Beck, J.S. and Newman, C.F. (1993) Hopelessness, depression, suicidal ideation and clinical diagnosis of depression. *Suicide and Life Threatening Behaviour*, 23, 139–145.

Barker, P. (2005) *Assessment in Practice*. In: Barker, P. (ed.) *Psychiatric and Mental Health Nursing: The craft of caring*. London: Hodder Arnold.

Carey, T.A. and Mullan R.J. (2004) What is Socratic Questioning? *Psychotherapy: Theory, Research, Practice, Training*, 41(3), 217–226.

Casement, P. (1985) *On Learning From the Patient*. London: Routledge.

Clark, G.I. and Egan, S.J . (2015) The Socratic method in cognitive behavioural therapy: A narrative review. *Cognitive Therapy and Research*, 39(6), 863–879.

Colley, G. (2009) Building Rapport – Customer Relations. www.evancarOliver.com. Accessed 25 January 2011.

Cutcliffe, J.R. and Stevenson, C. (2007) *Care of the Suicidal Person*. London: Churchill Livingston Elsevier.

Department of Health (2004) *The Ten Essential Shared Capabilities*. London: The Stationary Office.

Department of Health (2012) *Compassion in Practice: Nursing, Midwifery and Care Staff. Our Vision Our Strategy*. London: Department of Health.

Gladwell, M. (2005) *Blink: The power of thinking without thinking*. London: Penguin.

Goleman, D. (1996) *Working with Emotional Intelligence*. London: Bloomsbury.

Guthmann, E. (2005) The Allure: Beauty and an easy route to death have long made the Golden Gate Bridge a magnet for suicides. *The San Francisco Globe*.

Harrison, A. (2006) Self-harm and suicide prevention. In: Harrison, A. and Hart, C. (eds.) *Mental Health Care for Nurses: Applying mental health skills in the general hospital*. Oxford: Blackwell.

Hawton, K., Harriss, L. and Zahl, D. (2006) Deaths from all causes in a long term follow up study of 11,583 deliberate self-harm patients. *Psychological Medicine*, 36, 397–405.

Hoffman, W. and Wilson, T.D. (2010) Consciousness, Introspection, and the Adaptive Unconscious. In: Gawronski, B. and Payne, B.K. (eds.) *Handbook of Implicit Social Cognition: Measurement, Theory, and Applications*. New York: Guilford Press.

Hucker, S.J. (2005) Psychiatric Aspects of Risk Assessment. http://www.forensicpsychiatry.ca/risk/assessment.htm.

Kingdom, D. and Finn, M. (2006) *Tackling Mental Health Crisis*. London: Routledge.

Kukyen, W. (2006) Reasearch and evidence base in case formulation. In: Tarrier, N. (ed.) *Case Formulation in Cognitive Behaviour Therapy: The Treatment of Challenging and Complex Clinical Cases*. London: Routledge.

Leaviss, J. and Uttley, L. (2015) Psychotherapeutic benefits of compassion-focused therapy: an early systematic review. *Psychological Medicine*, 45(5), 927–45. DOI: 10.1017/S0033291714002141.

Linehan, M. (1993) *Cognitive-Behavioural Treatment of Borderline Personality Disorder*. New York: Guildford Press.

Luft, J. and Ingham, H. (1955) The Johari window, a graphic model of interpersonal awareness. *Proceedings of the western training laboratory in group development*. Los Angeles: UCLA.

Maden, T. (2007) *Treating violence: a guide to risk management in mental health*. Oxford University Press: Oxford.

Maden, T. (2013) Filmed Interview by Justin O'Brien. Unreleased.

McGranahan, T. (2004) *Treatment Risk Information System*. Unpublished Paper.

O'Brien, J. and Hart, C. (2013) Clinical Risk Assessment and Risk Management. London: South West London & St George's Mental Health NHS Trust.

Pearce, C.M., & Martin, G. (1993) Locus of control as an indicator of risk for suicidal behaviour among adolescents. *Acta Psychiatrica Scandinavica*, 88(6), 409–414.

Reynolds, B. (2003) Developing therapeutic one-to-one relationships. In: Barker, P. (ed.) *Psychiatric and Mental Health Nursing: The Craft of Caring*. London: Hodder Arnold.

Rotter, J.B. (1966). Generalized expectancies for internal versus external control of reinforcement. *Psychological monographs: General and applied*, 80(1), 1.

Smith, P. (1992) *The Emotional Labour of Nursing*. London: Macmillan Palgrave.

Stuart, G. (2005) Therapeutic nurse relationship. In: Stuart, G. and Laraira, M.T. (eds.), *Principles and Practice of Psychiatric Nursing*. St Louis: Elsevier Mosby.

Webster, C.D., Douglas, K.S., Eaves, D. and Hart, S.D. (1997) *HCR-20. Assessing Risk for Violence, Version 2*. Vancouver: Mental Health, Law and Policy Institute, Simon Fraser University.

Wilson, T. (2002) *Strangers To Ourselves: Discovering the Adaptive Consciousness*. Mass: Harvard University Press.

Part 4
Developing a risk formulation

Introduction

This was discussed briefly in 'Translating the assessment into a formulation' section of Part 2 (page 95). Case formulation is commonly used in psychology and psychiatry but less so in risk. As it is the bridge between an assessment and risk management plan, it should be viewed as an essential part of a seamless process.

The Royal College of Psychiatrists note a risk formulation:

> ...should take into account that risk is dynamic and, where possible, specify factors likely to increase the risk of dangerousness or those likely to mitigate violence, as well as signs that indicate increasing risk. [It] brings together an understanding of personality, history, mental state, environment, potential causes and protective factors, or changes in any of these.

This should aim to answer the following questions:

- How serious is the risk?
- Is the risk specific or general?
- How immediate is the risk?
- How volatile is the risk?
- What specific treatment, and which management plan, can best reduce the risk? (www. rcpsych.ac.uk.)

However, in this section we will also consider risk formulation from a patient's perspective.

The Five 'P's

In more in depth risk assessments, the same principles used in case formulation can be utilised in developing a risk formulation (known as 'The Five "P"s'). This involves considering any:

1. *Presenting problems*, i.e. what brought the person to your attention now?
2. *Precipitating factors*, i.e. what led up to the situation?
3. *Predisposing factors*, i.e. are there any factors, e.g. from their past or family history, that left them more vulnerable to this particular risk?

DOI: 10.4324/9781003171614-5

4. *Perpetuating factors*, i.e. what is likely to maintain their current situation and continue to leave them at risk?
5. *Protective factors*, i.e. what has enabled them to remain safe until this point?

The six point risk formulation model

In addition, you can consider:

- underpinning mechanisms or psychological processes and how these produce the presenting problems;
- obstacles to treatment;
- what might stop the person engaging in treatment.

The analysis of these different factors should then lead to a risk formulation which can help the clinician – and, therefore, the patient – conceptualise the patient's experience in terms of:

1. Who is at risk?
2. What, specifically, is the risk?
3. How are they at risk?
4. Where are they at risk?
5. When are they at risk?
6. Why are they at risk?

This can be broken down as follows:

Who is at risk?

This might seem obvious, but naming the person explicitly at risk is important, both for communication with other clinicians and also when thinking about care planning, particularly if aiming for a 'first person' care plan.

Key clinical tip

Identify and document:

- the person(s) at risk by name;
- if others are also at risk, if this is general or is a specific individual at risk;
- how someone will be warned if they, specifically, are at risk;
- the plan in place to protect individuals/groups.

What is the risk?

The aim is to identify, with the person and in the most explicit terms, the exact nature of the risk. If they say they wish to harm themselves, clarify what that means. Do they mean hurting themselves, or could this mean ending their life?

If the person is contemplating or planning suicide, that must be stated. It may mean asking, explicitly, "Do you want to end your life?" Some clinicians, especially those from a non mental health background, may find this challenging but it cannot be avoided. If the person has already been thinking about this, it is unlikely they'll find it difficult to answer and may even be relieved to be able to tell someone. Also, be specific. The person wanting to harm himself is *not* the same as wanting to kill themselves. This should be written in simple language, making sure everyone understands exactly what you mean.

Key clinical tip

Identify and document the risk. If there is more than one risk, name them all.

How would they be at risk?

If the risk is of suicide, how would they try to achieve this? By ligature? Self poisoning? More violent means? Asking about how they came to their decision will help you understand something of their thinking, e.g. if it has a specific meaning for them. It also leads to the question of how the methodology chosen relates to intent.

Key clinical tip

Identify and document:

- what they would do to place themselves at risk, e.g. attempt suicide by:
  - hanging;
  - self poisoning;
  - more violent means.
- if it has a specific meaning for them;
- how they chose the methodology and how it relates to intent.

<u>Where</u> is the person at risk?

This takes the assessor closer to the area of scenario planning, as the person may not be able to fully think through places they would be safe. However, they may be clear in their mind about places they are not safe. Looking back at Emma's case, being at home might increase the risk of self-harming behaviour because of the particularly difficult relationship with her mother at that time. In William's case, the significant thing might be because he is alone in his flat. For Oliver, the increase of his violence increases if he is in close proximity to people he believes are about to harm him. For someone in prison, it might be when they are in crowded areas of the prison, during association or 'freeflow'[i] if the risk is of violence. If the risk pertains to self-harm or suicide, it is likely to be greater when they are in their cell, especially if alone.

However, the risk might increase for someone if they are with certain people, e.g. someone who might offer them illicit substances that, in turn, increase the risk of impulsive behaviours.

Considering the different risk factors, you must also take account of the degree of collaboration. If away from clinicians and potential carers for any length of time, will they contact you if the risk increases? Are there things about the environment, e.g. the amount of stimulation, or potential and less predictable stressors over which the patient has limited or no control etc, that lead you to conclude the risk of remaining there is too great? In that case, do they need to be in a more secure environment? This includes considering the safety of a patient already in an acute psychiatric unit and whether that is suitable.

Consider what happens when someone leaves an environment in which they are safe and goes elsewhere, especially if it leaves them more exposed. For example, the person may feel calmer, safer, much less likely to act upon ideas about harming themselves in an Emergency Department. How will they manage when they leave there and return to the environment in which they were in when the crisis arose?

If a decision is made to place someone in an environment designed to be safe for them, e.g. a hospital ward, there needs to be a clear understanding that it is not just about having a physical environment in which the patient is safe but that the time they are there is used to prepare them to return to somewhere they were previously at risk.

Key clinical tip

Identify and document:

- where the person is safest and how that will be accommodated, e.g. if they have to be admitted to an inpatient unit or more secure environment, or away from other prisoners in a prison environment;
- places where the person is at greatest risk;
- which people might increase/decrease the risk;
- As much as possible, the degree of collaboration and less predictable risk factors or things that might change the risk over which the patient has limited or no control.

When is the person at risk?

This is slightly more complex than other headings in this section. When someone is at risk can be a point in time, e.g. now, tonight, the next day etc. But it can also allude to 'when something specific happens', the time of which is not yet determined.

If it's at some stage in the future this suggests something – and possibly something specific – would have to happen to increase the risk. What would that be? How does the person know this would increase the risk? Conversely, are they aware of anything that might decrease the risk?

Another dimension of the 'when?' question is situational: the person who says, "I have more thoughts of killing myself in the evening when I'm feeling particularly low." Or, "I cut myself when I'm on my own and stressed."

If the risk is immediate, i.e. happening now, a risk management plan needs to be put in place, including where the person will be safe. If the risk is likely to change in association with a specific but future event, the question is not just where the person will be safe at that time, but what can be done to try and either stop the potential triggering event or phenomena having the effect the person expects?

If the person acknowledges they were thinking of suicide or self-harm but no longer are, the key question is, 'what has changed?'

You need to be able to satisfy yourself about what, exactly, has changed for the person that now means they say they can behave in a safe manner. Moreover, you need to feel satisfied that this is a credible account. It is entirely natural to compose a narrative, retrospectively, to explain to ourselves why we did something or how a series of events occurred. This can vary as time goes on and is more likely to be altered to fit within our overall cognitive schema as we have more time to reflect. It can also feel very difficult for someone to have to tell a relative stranger about something that they now find very embarrassing, even ashamed. It is important, therefore, as a clinician to be clear the person is providing an accurate account of events, including their current vulnerability.

Another reason for any potential change in the person's presentation, now they have acted, could be that they have stopped ruminating, feel less physiologically aroused, less distressed and the suicidal impulse has reduced. This may offer you the opportunity to work with someone quite fruitfully but, if there is any ongoing denial of what happened, it is less likely.

It's also possible any perception the person has of feeling 'better' will be boosted by being out of the environment and/or situation which precipitated the act, which may contribute to a sense of being able to cope. All of this has to be built into a line of questioning that explores future coping and 'what if?' scenario planning. Another way of assessing the situation is, if possible, to check by tracking the story back, e.g. to paramedics, police, prison officers or family/carer's accounts of when the incident occurred.

Finally, you do have to consider whether or not the person is simply misleading you in the hope that they will be able to go away and make a further attempt to kill themself. Unless you are convinced something has happened to lessen the risk you should regard it as ongoing.

Key clinical tip

Identify and document:

- an immediate risk management plan if the risk is current;
- what might happen to increase the risk in the future;
- if the person will still be safe in their current location if the risk increases;
- *What has changed* for the person if they tell you the risk is apparently in the past and no longer current.

Why is the person at risk?

There can be numerous reasons the person may be at risk. These vary from the external, e.g. what is happening around them or what others are doing, to the internal e.g. their own thoughts and feelings. Most likely it will be a combination of both. Considering these factors can help with thinking about the likely effectiveness of any proposed risk management plan.

We have already looked at Joiner's Model and reasons why people develop suicidal ideas or think about self-harming behaviours. These are, though, generic. The important issue when assessing someone is to identify what it is about this person's experience that led them to this situation.

In Emma's case, discussion of her personal and family history revealed she has experienced significant trauma throughout her early years and into her teens. Indeed, from her account, she still suffered traumatic experiences within her relationship with her mother. If we go back to the suicidal crossroads diagram (Figure 1.10) we can see how events from her more distant past might have affected her resilience, made it difficult to develop coping strategies and an inability to adapt. More recent events, such as her anxiety about university and perceived problems with friends have triggered ruminations and emotional distress. This combination has left her vulnerable and, finding herself on a bridge, with the perception that her situation is hopeless and she could no longer cope, she jumped.

Key clinical tip

Identify and document:

- both external and internal factors, e.g.:
  - a change to the person's circumstances caused by a relationship breakup;
  - any mental disorder, such as depression;
  - any distressing ruminations and the impact on the person's emotional state;
  - any feelings of hopelessness, feeling trapped and/or lacking in choices;
- any events or responses that exacerbate or minimise the situation;
- your understanding of the process of how external factors and the person's emotional/psychological state are affecting the risk;
- anything the person and clinical team can do to influence it and reduce the risk.

In the case of William, a patient who has attempted suicide and is still experiencing suicidal ideation, the risk formulation might be written as follows:

William is a 35-year-old man who took an overdose of 18 Paracetamol 500mg tablets with the intention of ending his life, alone in his flat last night. He took the tablets after ruling out other means, such as throwing himself in front of a fast train. He thought it would prove fatal and told his family he would not be home that evening to try and avoid discovery. He was found by his ex-partner, Kelly, who had come to the flat to collect some personal belongings, believing he'd be out. She called an ambulance.

William's suicide attempt followed his difficulties coping with his father's death a year ago, after a long illness, and his recent separation from Kelly. He was also made redundant from his job in information technology and has had financial problems following cuts in his benefits, causing him to worry he will lose his flat.

William says he has "complicated relationships" with his mother and brother, has few friends and finds it hard to confide in others. Although describing his relationship with Kelly as "difficult", he "became dependent on her" and "can't go on"

*because of how he feels without her in his life. Struggling to cope with mounting
stress, he's been drinking more and described "crowded thoughts running in circles" which are too much for him. He's stopped doing things that acted as protective factors.*

*William has had depressive symptoms, e.g. poor sleep, loss of appetite, trouble
concentrating and not enjoying things he used to, for approximately six weeks. He
sees no hope for the future and thinks no one would miss him if he were dead. He
sees no way out of his situation and regrets surviving his suicide attempt.*

*He is still ruminating on his situation, feeling very distressed and having ideas of
ending his life.*

The importance of this structural approach following the identification of risk is that
it then makes it easier to develop a risk management plan to address these elements
(see Part 5), as well as forming an accessible and easily understood communication to
colleagues.

This should all be documented and linked to the risk management plan. In William's
case this would be:

Immediate:

- helping him stay away from the means to end his life;
- helping him identify what makes things worse for him and what makes things better;
- helping him to access his coping strategies problem solving techniques and protective
  factors again;
- breaking into his ruminations by helping him distract and ground himself, then starting to challenge his negative thoughts etc;
- helping him regulate his emotions, particularly lessening his distress;
- treating his depressive symptoms.

Table 4.1 Formulating the risk

Who is at risk:	William.
What is the risk:	Suicide. He ingested an overdose of 18 Paracetamol tablets and is still experiencing suicidal ideation.
How is William at risk:	Taking a further overdose. Though he may try to use another method if he hasn't access to tablets, as he considered different methods prior to the overdose.
Where is the risk:	When he is alone, particularly back at his flat.
When is William at risk:	Now (currently) but exacerbated by any increase in his ruminations and stress levels.
Why is William at risk:	• His emotional and psychological reaction to separation from his girlfriend suggest poor resilience. • Strong depressive features following the death of his father, financial worries and the potential loss of his accommodation. • He is unable to access his usual coping strategies and there is an absence of current protective factors in the form of his relationship with his brother and mother. • He feels trapped, hopeless and cannot see any other way out of his situation.

Once his situation has stabilised:

- helping him with practical issues such as his finances and accommodation.

Once he is in the recovery phase:

- longer term, addressing his lack of resilience.

The patient's perception – a risk formulation from the patient

All of this reflects a clinical view of the persons situation, risk(s) and potential solutions. The patient may have a very different view of things. Even the collaborative person may formulate their situation and associated risks quite differently. Indeed, working towards a shared understanding of the situation and a shared formulation is key to collaborative working.

Table 4.2 demonstrates how someone may have a completely different view of their situation and risk from the clinicians trying to work with them. In this case, the focus is Oliver. The discrepancy here can be largely attributed to his psychotic disorder. However, Emma (in case study 3) and even William (in case study 1) would likely provide a different risk formulation to that of the clinicians working with them.

Space prevents using the same model for all three but, looking at Table 4.2, as it speculates on how Oliver might respond to questions, it is easy to imagine the answers Emma and William might give.

Table 4.2 Contrasting a Clinical Risk Formulation with a Patient's Risk Formulation

	As the clinician may understand the issues	As Oliver may understand the issues
Who is affected by the phenomena?	Is it the patient alone? Is someone else at risk from the patient? Be specific – who is at risk?	Is it the same person(s) as we think it is? If there is a discrepancy, why?
	"Oliver's psychotic experience puts Daniel and members of the nursing team at risk, particularly Ola and Jane."	*"I'm affected. They're putting stuff into me and threatening me."*
What are the presenting phenomena?	What, specifically, is happening? Is it a risk of suicide, self-harm, dangerousness to others? What led to the change?	The person may see the issue as needing to escape, or find relief from, unmanageable distress rather than the risk behaviours being a problem. What happened that they are now more at risk of acting?
	"Oliver is psychotic (experiencing auditory hallucinations and delusional beliefs) and presents as a risk to Daniel and staff because he believes they are doing things to him and pose a threat."	*"Dan's able to put things inside me. Jane and Ola have been talking about me. They're going to do something to me."*

Why is it happening?	Be clear if it is mental health related. In what way? Is it a change in the person's mental state, situation etc? Are the risk behaviours occurring in a certain context, e.g. recent discharge from hospital, increased hopelessness etc?	Does the person understand other people's concern? Do they believe it is related to their mental health? What do they see as the cause of things happening to them? Has the specific risk occurred because of something internal or because of others and, if the latter, what they are doing?
	"Oliver is in hospital because of another severe psychotic breakdown several months ago but also has a history of violence when not experiencing any symptoms and has been formally diagnosed as having anti social personality traits. He only takes his medication intermittently and is under a lot of stress. There have been disputes with Daniel. The more threatened he feels, the greater the likelihood of him reacting in a dangerous way."	*"There's nothing wrong with me. I understand what's going on. They're doing this because they know I'm special. They have no respect and think I'm weak. They don't like me and Dan is affecting the staff, to turn them against me."*
How is it affecting the person?	What has happened to the person's behaviour? Has it changed the identified risk(s)?	Does the person recognise there has been any change? Do they have a sense that there is any risk attached to their behaviour?
	"He has been spending more time in his room, isolated, playing music on his headphones. He is more irritable, getting into arguments with other patients, particularly Daniel, and has made threats to him and staff members, Ola and Jane. His sleep has deteriorated, he appears agitated and hypervigilant at times. *He is very sensitive to what's said to him, less able to rationalise his situation and what is happening around him and it is probable he would respond violently if he felt particularly threatened."*	*"I'm being constantly hassled and disrespected. I have to watch out for people looking at me for signs of weakness, planning, setting me up. Dan's been doing it and now he's got nurses in on it. I've tried staying away from them, in my room, playing music to shut them out but it isn't working. I can't sleep. I can't think properly. I'm not safe."*
Where is it happening?	Is there a specific context, place or situation in which the risk occurs?	Is there anywhere specific the person feels less safe? Do they do anything to lessen the risk in certain situations or avoid particular places?
	"Times he is with a lot of other patients, e.g. mealtimes, OT sessions, when with Daniel. There are other times when he seeks out staff, seeming agitated and stressed for no obvious reason and can be irritable and argumentative with staff."	*"Anywhere outside my room but even in there they can get at me. They gang up on me when I go for my meals and the nurses might be giving me different tablets, not the ones the doctors prescribed. When Dan is talking with staff I know they're seeing if this is the right time to get me."*

Table 4.2 (Continued)

When is it happening?	Is there a specific time at which the risk occurs? Is the risk current, i.e. occurring now, or potential, i.e. in the future or past?	Does the person share an understanding of risk at the time clinicians view it as occurring? Do they worry about what may happen in the future? If they say the risk was in the past, what has changed that it is no longer a risk?
	"The risk is current. There doesn't seem to be a time of day when it's worse but it heightens when he's in high stress situations such as around Daniel or lots of patients."	*"It's happening all the time."*
What purpose does it serve?	Are the risk behaviours a coping mechanism, e.g. self-harm, or a means of escaping an intolerable situation/feeling, e.g. suicide?	Does the person perceive what clinicians see as a 'risk' having any benefit?
	"Oliver feels the need to protect himself but it also seems to be a way of trying to stop staff talking to him about how his psychosis has affected him, the hardship and losses he has experienced in his life."	*"I have to protect myself."*
What triggered the risk (or were the precipitants)?	What changed in the person's life that started the risk behaviours or increased the sense of risk?	Is the person aware of issues that relate to his risk?
	"Oliver's keyworker left the community team caring for him. He was subsequently discharged from services and stopped taking his medication, suffering a psychotic relapse. He had no insight into his illness and was brought into hospital under the Mental Health Act. There have been several incidents of assaultive behaviour in the context of his psychosis."	*"I got brought into hospital because I upset one of the doctors. They keep lying about stuff they say I've done and saying I'm ill. But I'm not. They don't understand what people try to do to me or what is happening."*
What factors maintain or perpetuate it?	Is it clear what keeps it going? This might be high levels of stress, lack of support, non adherence to medication, substance misuse etc.	Is the person aware of issues that relate to his risk?
	"Oliver finds it very difficult to trust and talk to anyone about his problems When he's stressed he increases his use of illicit substances, doesn't think he has a mental disorder and stops taking his medication. More paranoid on the ward, he believes others are going to harm him."	*"They know I have special powers. They're against me and they're going to do something, but I don't know what it is."*
Are there any predisposing factors?	Is there a family history? Is there a history of developmental problems etc.?	Are there any historic reasons the person cites as having influenced her/his current situation?

	"His father had a psychotic disorder and his early life was marred by family trauma. He was the victim of domestic violence and possibly sexual abuse."	*"People have always been against me. My dad was no good and mum brought weirdos into the home. She never looked after me properly."*
What are the protective factors?	These might be related to family, beliefs, support mechanisms, e.g. existing mental health services, coping mechanisms, avoidance techniques etc.	The person may share your understanding of these. However, they may also have other factors that are important to them which you may think harmful, e.g. certain relationships, behaviours, substance misuse, non adherence to treatment, contact with services.
	"There are none at the moment. Mum used to be supportive but hasn't seen Oliver for some months."	*"Staying away from staff who want to damage me. Being out of hospital and being able to get on with my life."*
What makes it worse?	Are there specific things the person does or that happen that increase the risk?	Does the person regard the things clinicians see as exacerbating the situation as making it worse?
	"Not taking his medication. Psychotic symptooms i.e. delusional beliefs and hallucinations. Stress. Increased contact with Daniel and exposure to large groups of patients. Lack of sleep and ruminating on his own psychotic perceptions. Using illicit substances."	*"It's not me. It's them."*
What makes it better?	Are there specific things the person does or that happen that decrease the risk?	Does the person perceive any benefit from change? Do they view things clinicians view as beneficial as harmful, e.g. medication?
	"Medication would be a major help for Oliver now. It has worked very effectively in the past. He would also benefit from a specific plan to address the risk of him assaulting others, talking about his ideas, with cognitive behavioural techniques such as Socratic questioning, behavioural plans and motivational interviewing being used."	*"I'm not taking anything you want to give me. I know you want to put stuff inside me. Everything will be fine when I'm out of here."*

If you've worked through a formulation in this way, contrasting the patient's views with that of the clinician, it's possible to see not only the plan you want to implement to address the risk but also any areas of disagreement between yourself and the patient, recognising that these will likely be obstacles to treatment and helping the person stay safe. Why would Oliver agree to medication to treat a disorder he doesn't believe he has and which he believes will be harmful? Why would he agree to leave himself in a situation where he feels vulnerable and at direct threat from others?

Bridging the gap between the clinician's understanding of the situation and Oliver's is necessary if he is going to be successfully treated. In this case, given the immediacy and seriousness of the risks identified, this will almost certainly involve treating him against his will and imposing restrictions upon him during the early stages of treatment. As that progresses, the crucial issue will be how successfully the team can find a way into working with Oliver that eventually gains his trust, collaboration and helps him re-interpret his situation in such a way that he no longer poses a threat to others or himself.

Note

i This is when prisoners or residents are unlocked from their cells and allowed to move around certain areas of the prison freely alongside others from their landing or wing/houseblock.

References and selected bibliography

Department of Health (2007) *Best Practice in Managing Risk: Principles and evidence for best practice in the assessment and management of risk to self and others in mental health services.* London: Department of Health.

Royal College of Psychiatrists. Formulating Risk. https://www.rcpsych.ac.uk/members/supporting-your-professional-development/assessing-and-managing-risk-of-patients-causing-harm/formulating-risk.

Part 5
Managing risk

Introduction

There are, essentially, two basic rules for managing risk. Firstly, hope for the best but plan for the worst (Maden, 2007). Secondly, always aim for the least restrictive option when working with patients but balance that with consideration for the safety of the patient and/or others and be prepared to be as restrictive as is necessary.

In this part of the *Pocket Guide*, we will consider the underlying principles and practice of risk management and the use of the information gathered at assessment, developed into a formulation, to progress to risk management with a goal of risk reduction (see Table 5.1). While we will be focusing on risk to self and/or others, the same principles can be applied to the management of any other kind of risk, e.g. the person who is vulnerable to exploitation etc. This involves:

* maximising potentially protective factors;
* minimising exacerbating factors;
* acknowledging potential outcomes – and being clear about the potentially best *and* worst;
* ensuring that clinicians given the responsibility for managing the risk also have the *authority* to manage risks identified, e.g.:

  * making clinical decisions, including adjusting the risk management plan in response to – and ideally in anticipation of – dynamic change in relation to the person's risk;
  * In community settings this means the staff who have risk assessed the patient should be able to admit them if necessary, or utilise more intensive home visits, rather than decisions being made by clinicians or managers who have not seen the patient or been involved in the assessment;
  * in inpatient areas, this involves those directly managing the risk determining levels of 'observation' or available support and other issues necessary to help the patient and others remain safe, if there is a clear case for how they will be used and the benefits;

* managing the environment around the person as much as is practical.

However, it is important to remind ourselves that not every risk can or should be 'managed'. This is the case if there is not a mental health component to someone's behaviour, e.g. if someone becomes violent when drunk or having taken illicit substances, or is threatening violence or other criminal acts as a means of achieving something to their

DOI: 10.4324/9781003171614-6

advantage or their own pleasure. Clinicians are sometimes drawn into trying to 'manage' such situations – very rarely with any success.

Nor does even the best assessment allow you to predict the future. It does allow the clinician to develop a coherent, rational plan to address the most obvious or likely risks as well as those already clearly identified. The concept of proactive, enabling, or thera-peutic, risk management is discussed below (page 207).

At this stage it is, once again, worth reminding ourselves that the best we can achieve is to minimise risk. We can never completely eliminate it and, ultimately, the only person who can maintain their safety is the person themselves. The key role of the clinician is to do everything possible to assist them in doing that.

Mental capacity

We cannot explore in detail here issues of capacity and consent and you should famil-iarise yourself with local and national guidance and policy in this area. The Mental Ca-pacity Act (2005), Section 2(1), emphasises that healthcare professionals should assume people 16-years-old and over are competent to make decisions about their care unless there is evidence to the contrary. The Act goes on to state that a person 'lacks capacity in relation to a matter if *at the material time* he is unable to make a decision for himself in relation to the matter' due to 'impairment' or 'disturbance in the functioning *of the mind or brain*' [my italics].

The essential issues to consider are:

1. Is the person able to understand the information you are giving them and the issues being discussed?
2. Can they retain that information?
3. Can they weigh up the information and arrive at a decision?
4. Have they been able to consider all the options available?
5. Do they understand the implications of the decision and its likely consequences?

Few could ever agree with an argument put forward by an individual that they had the right to kill someone else. Nor would most people feel they couldn't or wouldn't take any action to stop them doing it. However, clinicians often find the issue of capacity more complex when considering the case of the suicidal patient. Ethical, professional and moral issues – not always assisted by professional codes of practice – come into play here, but when thinking about the individual's immediate safety, our duty of care should always lead us to provide adequate safeguards, even if they don't concur with the person's wishes, while recognising that capacity is a fluid concept, often difficult to assess and liable to fluctuation.

It is useful to have a solid grounding in the ethics of decision-making and the suicidal patient but this can often feel very distant to the clinician sitting in the room with some-one intent on taking their life. It is thus necessary to pay very close attention to every-thing the person says, weighing up their internal logic against your own, hopefully, more objective view.

For example, the person may be expressing feelings of hopelessness about their fu-ture despite some obvious options for treatment, as well as evidence that they would benefit from these. In addition, they may be saying they're unable to solve their prob-lems when they would have been able to do so in the recent past. They may also say everyone will be better off if they are dead, when you have already been alerted by relatives who are very concerned for the person. In such circumstances, it would be difficult to argue the person has the ability to weigh up information and consider all the options available.

Even someone with a terminal illness, demanding the right to end their life might be seeking to do so based on incomplete or incorrect information, fuelled by their own perception of their situation, e.g. a patient wanting to end their life because they fear an imminent, insufferably painful death when, in fact, their prognosis is for several years of relatively good health and who has the ongoing support of an experienced, skilled palliative care team.

There are other potential complications. Ayre et al. (2017) put a compelling argument that, for patients with borderline personality disorder (also known as emotionally unstable personality disorder): 'in some cases the decision to refuse [life saving treatment] *per se* may simply be a manifestation of the disorder, rather than a carefully considered wish to die'. In other cases, they suggest refusing treatment, or help, can be 'a disturbed form of engagement ... rather than an effort to disengage'. They support this latter view by quoting the case of B v. Croydon Health Authority, where:

> *A young woman with BPD was starving herself to the point where enforced nasogastric feeding was considered. Lord Justice Hoffman wrote in his judgment that he found it difficult to conclude that the patient had capacity, despite her seeming to have a good understanding of the risks and options. It was this that made him question whether her choice was truly autonomous, because, while being able to make cogent and articulate statements about her wishes, it was hard for him to deem someone capacitous when she is "crying inside for help but unable to break out of the routine of punishing herself".*

Moreover, there is some evidence emerging from neuro-imaging which has revealed significant brain abnormalities in people experiencing suicidal ideas, including differences in those with suicidal ideation and clinical depression and those who are suicidal but not depressed. Post-mortem studies have also revealed neurobiological dysfunction related to suicide independent of major depression. There appear to be three characteristics which differentiate people with depression who are suicidal from people with depression who are not. Those who are suicidal are more likely to show:

1. a sensitivity to particular life events reflecting signals of defeat, based on attentional biases ('perceptual popout'). This leads to an involuntary hypersensitivity to stimuli which the individual perceives signals their 'loser' status;
2. a sense of being 'trapped', related to insufficient capacity to solve problems, commonly of an interpersonal or social nature;
3. the absence of rescue factors, mediated by deficient prospective cognitive processes and leading to feelings of hopelessness (Van Heeringen and Maruia, 2003).

This seems to tie in with cognitive theories and research by Williams et al. (2005) and others into what lies behind suicidal ideation, which identify several key factors:

1. **Entrapment** – the inability or perceived inability to escape from 'an aversive environment after one has suffered a defeat, loss or humiliation'.

2. **The arrested flight model** – there are three elements to this:

   a. sensitivity to cues that signal defeat or humiliation. The person may misinterpret even relatively neutral events, such as the expression on others' faces and chance comments, or view minor issues such as making simple mistakes as complete failure;
   b. an 'overwhelming feeling of *needing to escape*; a sense of being *unable to escape*'. This seems to arise from deficits in interpersonal problem solving as well as over-generalised memory;
   c. the sense that '*this state of affairs will continue indefinitely*', which contributes to the feeling of hopelessness so often described by those experiencing suicidal ideation (italics in original) (Williams et al., 2005).

Both of these areas of research suggest that, indeed, there are some profound changes in the functioning of the mind and brain.

Exploring options for treatment with people who are psychotic, pose a risk to others and lack capacity or are reluctant to accept treatment, Maden (2007) has argued cogently that all aspects of the individual's capacity have to be explored in depth and clinical teams should adopt the maxim of treating when in doubt, on the basis that people have the right to be treated and, despite any potential difficulties it may create in the relationship with the individual, the safest option is often the wisest. The same principles could be said to apply to the potentially suicidal person. Of course, these decisions don't have to be made in isolation by a clinician. While capacity is often best assessed by someone who knows the patient well, consulting with a colleague or even colleagues who might then further assess the person is good practice if there is any doubt.

While wanting to offer the least restrictive option, this has be balanced with a risk management plan that has sufficient restrictions to provide the safest option for a person lacking capacity, unable or unwilling to cooperate and posing a risk to themself or others. Greater levels of caution must be exercised when there is a more serious level of potential risk. This might include the use of the Mental Health Act 1983 (as amended in 2007) and restrictive settings such as inpatient wards, Psychiatric Intensive Care Units (PICUs) or secure units. In a prison setting, this may mean initiating constant observation, moving the person to an inpatient unit (if available in the prison or even a secure bed in an outside hospital), or considering the use of the prison's care and separation unit if the risk is one of violence to others

Negotiating and writing a care plan for the purposes of risk management

Care plans are often the source of a great deal of confusion. How should they be written (and by whom)? What is their purpose? How long should they be in place? The care plans highlighted in the *Pocket Guide* are not long term or the type that feature in the Care Planning Approach (CPA) documentation. These are short term, focused on specific risk issues and designed to be evaluated and adapted as a response to small but important changes, in the context of risk either increasing or decreasing.

They follow a relatively simple formula: identifying a problem or need, an objective to resolve that, with specific interventions to directly address the risks identified, which should be followed by the patient and clinical staff (see Table 5.1). The risk management plan, wherever possible, should be created collaboratively with the patient, even though the clinician may write the plan itself, to give it a consistent structure. Even if the patient is non collaborative and a management plan has to be written, the plan should be shared

Table 5.1 A framework for a risk management plan

Identify who is at risk, naming the person(s) involved or at risk, e.g. William wants to kill himself etc; Oliver wants to assault Daniel etc.	Is the risk actual (immediate) or potential? E.g., something will have to happen to increase the risk or likelihood of the person acting.
Clear identification and description of the risk, in the simplest, most easily understandable terms.	How willing is the person to collaborate? Will this be an agreed care plan or a management plan that has to be imposed on the individual?
Name the desired outcome (objective) directly related to the specific problem identified.	If the person is collaborating, the objective would be that they will keep themself safe. If there is no collaboration it would be that the team will work to keep the person safe.
List the interventions required to achieve the objective.	Maximise potentially protective factors and minimise exacerbating factors.
Who, specifically, will do what to manage the risk?	• The patient. • The primary nurse/keyworker. • Others from the MDT.
A time frame for addressing the situation/ behaviours.	This should be short enough to adapt the plan according to its effectiveness, i.e. a few days only.

with the patient and communicated with the team, other clinicians and agencies that need to be aware of it.

In Table 5.2, we can see how the specific risks identified in William's risk formulation can be addressed in a risk management plan. Table 5.3 then demonstrates the structure for a care plan and the principles underpinning it.

Different organisations have their own way of writing care plans, usually determined by their electronic records system and its framework. Any difficulties in electronic record systems, particularly in providing a simple pathway from assessment to formulation to care plan, constitutes a clear organisational risk which should be addressed as soon as possible. The problems sometimes include care plans not being readily accessible, so often not read or followed up on by team members.

Teams should both familiarise themselves with the particular structural frameworks of their system in as much detail as possible but also be aware of its limitations. The aim is for risk management plans to be accessible, practical, easy to understand and have a consistent, coherent structure for writing them.

Even when someone is feeling very distressed and/or disturbed, it is usually possible to have a conversation about what they want or, preferably, need to help them at that time.

If, for any reason, the person is unable to work with you to keep themself and others safe, this *has* to be pro-actively addressed. It is one of the very few times that you, in collaboration with the rest of the clinical team, should impose a care plan. It may also raise safeguarding issues. Imposing a plan will almost always happen in an inpatient environment or PICU and, in such cases, it is important that the ownership of the problem is with the team and most particularly the ward nurses, as it is the nurses who will spend the majority of time with the person and may have to physically intervene to maintain everyone's safety. Therefore, the interventions should remain with the nurses and other team members but be specific, clear and with the single objective of keeping the person and others safe. If this does require a management plan, i.e. something imposed on the patient against their will, it is necessary to ensure one intervention is to continually assess the patient's capacity and willingness to collaborate so that a negotiated care plan can be developed at the earliest time.[i]

Below are two examples of safety care plans, one for an inpatient setting, one for the community and a risk management plan for a non collaborative patient. As well as care plans being shaped by electronic record systems, particular organisations may also have models or templates for the writing of care plans, Nonetheless, it is useful to look at some simple principles that make the plan easy to write, understand and implement, as well as measurable and straightforward to evaluate.

Principles of care planning

The concept of a care plan is to provide the clinician and patient with an agreement about:

- a clear problem or need *expressed in behavioural terms*;
- a proposed solution (the objective *expressed in a change in behaviour*);
- the interventions to make it possible to achieve the objective and who will do what for each intervention. This involves:
  - what will be discussed:
  - how often the discussion will take place;
  - how long the discussions will last;
  - practical steps to lessen the risk;
  - the overall time frame over which the work will take place (Ritter, 1989).

The emphasis on expressing both the problem or need in behavioural terms and objective as a change in behaviour is that this can then be measured. In its simplest form, is a person who is planning to end their life still alive when the time comes to evaluate the care plan? Has the person who was behaving in a violent manner stopped being violent? Has the person cutting themself stopped cutting? If that is the case, the care plan can be seen to have been successful. Similarly, the interventions should describe observable events, e.g. meeting for a specific time on a specific number of occasions, making a list about specific things, carrying out a specific activity. Through doing this, the clinician will access particular emotions and thoughts and, if the care plan is written properly, that will be far easier than vague notions such as 'monitor the patient's mental state', or 'allow the patient to vent...'

It is essential that a safety care plan is about **one** problem or need, which is the identified risk. This should never be conflated with other issues. This is true even when the risk is associated, for example, with psychosis. In an instance like this there should be a care plan for treating the psychosis, e.g. by the administration of medication etc. and a separate plan for addressing the risk issues.

While all plans for patients should be recovery oriented, a care plan (as opposed to a management plan that must be imposed on a patient for safety reasons) should also be:

- person-centred, coming from the person's perspective;
- written in simple language and, if not using the person's own words exactly, retaining their spirit while having a structure that will enable other clinicians to understand and use it in a consistent fashion, and for it to be evaluated.

A structure for writing care plans

The starting point must be a conversation between yourself and the patient. As has been emphasised throughout, the goal of the assessment is to identify any risks affecting the person you are assessing. However, you should also be attempting to do this in such a way that you arrive not only at a shared understanding of those risks but also potential solutions. Several of the clinical examples already shown demonstrated ways in which this might be achieved.

Explicitly naming the problem allows an equally explicit statement about the solution or objective. These components of a plan are often easier than working through who will do what to meet that objective, in terms of interventions. However, careful listening to the person will usually offer clues (see clinical example 24).

Clinical Example 24:   Negotiating a safety care plan in a community setting

Clinician: Thanks for that. Is there anything we've missed or that you want to add?

William: No. That's everything.

Clinician: I know this has been a difficult conversation at times but we've covered a lot of ground. I want to turn now to how Sarah and I can help you stay safe.

William: I told you; I'll be okay.

Clinician: I'd like to think that. But you've described your thoughts about killing yourself, even how you'd do it. That doesn't sound okay to me.

William: [*Silence*]

Clinician: Earlier on, I touched on some ideas–

William: I'm not going into hospital. I told you that.

Clinician: Yes, you did. But my concern is that you have another night when you can't sleep, the thoughts going round and round in your head, and you can't switch them off, have a panic attack–

William: That won't happen.

Clinician: It could. And you might do what you've been thinking about: taking some tablets. I want to discuss some quite specific things to help you keep yourself safe.

William: Do you think I'm still thinking about killing myself or I'd do anything like that after talking with you?

Clinician: [*Pause*] I'm not sure. Do you?

William: [*Long pause*] What about if I come and see you regularly?

Clinician: How would that help, do you think?

William: It's helped me today. I feel like I've cleared my head a bit [*pause*]. I've also realised maybe I can be helped. I don't know... I felt really helpless, like there was no way out...

Clinician: And now?

William:	Well, if I can sleep, like you said, that'll help me feel better. I can stay with my mum 'til my brother gets back. I don't want to worry her though…
Clinician:	But you said she is worried about you.
William:	Yeah. Now I wish I'd listened to her and James and tried to get some help earlier. Or even said more to Dr Patterson when I saw her at the surgery.
Clinician:	So coming in to talk with us would help. And getting more sleep.
William:	Yes.
Clinician:	What else? You did mention there were things you used to do when you were feeling down before that helped you.
William:	I know. When I'm like this I have to make a plan for the day. Write it down and stick to it.
Clinician:	Will you be able to do that?
William:	Now I will be. I don't know why I didn't think of it before.
Clinician:	What sort of things will you do?
William:	Go for walks. I always used to go for two long walks a day with the dog but I stopped. Making sure I have a bath every day. Eating at set times. I don't know why, but all that helps. You said about making lists of things that help me and stuff that drags me down. I'll do that.
Clinician:	Would you be able to do that before you come in to see me next time? [*William nods*] Sometimes it's useful to write down how you're feeling at different times of the day and why that might be.
William:	Um, I said, didn't I? Like feeling worse in the evening, when I start thinking a lot about Kelly not being there.
Clinician:	Yes, so the early evening might be a good time to go for a walk…

[*Later in the interview*]

Clinician:	Okay, while you and Sarah were talking, I've made a note of where we've got to. As I said earlier, we try and write these plans or agreements in a certain way but I've tried to capture what we were talking about. Would you take a look at how I've written it and see what you think?
William:	[*Reads the care plan*] Yes, it's okay.
Clinician:	The most important thing is, do you think it's manageable for you?
William:	Even talking about it has helped. I don't know. It's given me something to think about and I've got things I can do.
Clinician:	So we'll see you tomorrow and we'll also come to see you on Thursday. After that, we'll review whether we still need to meet daily.
William:	Yeah.

Clinician:	And you have our number, in case you need to get in touch in between meeting up.
William:	Uh huh.
Clinician:	What would you do if you felt things were getting on top of you and you can't cope? If you might do something to harm yourself?
William:	Well, I'd ring you or come down to the health centre. And if it was at night–
Clinician:	Which it might be–
William:	Then I'd ring that crisis line number or I could call James.
Clinician:	And it's okay for us to ring James and talk with him?
William:	I think it would help. You know, even though we're close, it would be difficult for me to tell him some of this stuff straight out.
Clinician:	Okay. If you felt really bad, you could go to A&E as well.
William:	I told you, I don't want to do that, because I'll end up seeing some doctor I don't know and they'll want to admit me to hospital. Anyway, I'm getting rid of all the tablets in the house and you'll only be bringing me a day's worth at a time.
Clinician:	I want to keep coming into A&E as an option, because at least we'll know you're safe.
William:	I'll be honest. I'd have to really be feeling desperate. And, anyway, you said that the crisis team could come out if I needed them.
Clinician:	Yes, they can, but I have to be honest as well. It can take a while. But we can let the mental health team who work in A&E know you might need to go there. They'll be able to read about everything we've talked about today so you won't have to explain it all over again. And you'll be somewhere safe.
William:	[*Silence, then nods*]
Clinician:	There's one last thing I need to discuss with you.
William:	Look, I'm really tired…
Clinician:	I'm sorry. This is important though.
William:	Okay.
Clinician:	Supposing something happens you're not expecting, like you see Kelly–
William:	[*Interrupts*] I won't see Kelly. That won't happen.
Clinician:	I don't mean intentionally, necessarily. Suppose you just see her in the street?
William:	[*Silence*]
Clinician:	Would you tell me what you're thinking about?
William:	[*Pause*] I was picturing it… seeing her… how I miss her, what I'd say…
Clinician:	You sound really sad.
William:	I… yeah… I am.
Clinician:	[*Sits silently*]

William:	[*Sighs*] I'm okay. Yeah. Go on.
Clinician:	[*Nods*] It's important we think about anything unexpected that might throw you off balance or you might struggle to cope with.
William:	[*Sighs*] Like what?
Clinician:	Does anything come to mind?
William:	No. Genuinely. I can't think of anything.
Clinician:	What about another bill coming in through the post? A phone call, bad news about something? And you think about giving the team a call but the thoughts of killing yourself come back and are stronger than you feel able to cope with? You remember we talked earlier about how people in your situation can find it difficult to solve problems or work their way through situations they normally would, and then you can feel trapped, with no way out?
William:	Yeah. I know that feeling only too well.
Clinician:	That's why I want to keep something like the A&E option open. As a last resort. You only have to ring 999 and let a paramedic in through the door.
William:	You worry too much. [*Smiles*]
Clinician:	[*Smiles back*]
William:	Okay. But I don't think I'll need it if you bring me those sleeping tablets. And you were saying the anti-depressants the GP gave me will start working in a few more days.
Clinician:	Well, more like a week or so. But it feels like we have got a plan.
William:	Yeah. It's helpful. I didn't think it would be but… yeah.

Example of a safety care plan written for a patient in the community

In clinical example 24, William and the clinicians have been through a thorough assessment. The clinicians have developed a risk formulation and discussed, with William, ways in which he might keep himself safe and their role in that while he avoids going into hospital. This is how the plan might read, with the clinician using William's own words and ideas to write it in the first person, i.e. from William's perspective:

Problem:
Over the last week, I have been thinking about killing myself in my flat.

Objective:
Over the next three days I will keep myself safe in my flat and when I'm out.

Interventions

I will:

1. Meet each day for the next three days, for 45 minutes, with John or Sarah to talk about how I'm coping and how safe I feel.

2. Make a list of things that used to help me when I felt depressed and had ideas about harming myself.
3. Make a list of things that make me feel worse and things that make me feel better now.
4. Bring the lists in with me for my next appointment and discuss it with John and Sarah.
5. Write a plan each day to give me a routine and follow it.
6. Go for a walk twice a day, lasting at least 30 minutes, once at lunchtime and once in the evening.
7. Use the distraction techniques I discussed with John and Sarah when my thoughts are stuck and negative or I'm feeling more stressed.
8. Get in touch with Mum and James each day to let them know what I'm doing and ask for help if I need it.
9. Contact John, Sarah or the team if I feel unsafe or am worried that I might harm myself. If it's after the team have finished work, I'll contact the crisis team or ring for an ambulance to take me to A&E.
10. Take the sleeping tablets and anti-depressant tablets as prescribed.

My nurses will:

1. Meet me each day, for 45 minutes, to talk about how I'm coping, if my coping strategies are working and how to solve any problems I am having.
2. Review how safe I feel and any thoughts about killing or hurting myself.
3. Discuss my lists with me and how I can use them to help myself stay safe.
4. Check I'm following my plan each day and sticking to my routine.
5. Get in touch with James to let him know what's been happening and make sure he feels okay to help.
6. Be available to meet me urgently if I feel unsafe or am worried that I might harm myself. Let the crisis team and A&E team know I might need to get in touch in the evening and give them a copy of this care plan.
7. Give my sleeping tablets and anti-depressants to me each day.

In the above example, William is an active participant in the care planning process. The clinician, John, writes the plan in a way that captures William's words and what he is prepared to do, though he was very assertive with him about keeping the option of using the A&E Department open in case of an unforeseen emergency. Whether or not he would use that option is uncertain but he has agreed to everything else, so the clinicians are working on the basis of there being sufficient interventions to help William remain safe and an increased likelihood he'd contact the A&E Department if the team are aware of his situation.

In not admitting him to hospital, there is an element of proactive, or enabling, risk management (see below) but this plan sits clearly within the essential principles of the recovery approach, using the least restrictive option , while being practical and clinically sound – with a contingency plan incorporated as part of the overall package. The structure of the care plan is detailed in Table 5.2.

The simplicity of the care plan is, hopefully, apparent. Though the interventions are detailed (and the detail is necessary as it addresses specific deficits William has identified), the language is straightforward. There is no jargon. It could be followed by anyone if either John or Sarah were unavailable. Were William to need to contact the crisis team, it would

Table 5.2 Structuring a care plan

Identifying the problem	Setting an objective to resolve the problem
Concerned person (whose problem is it?)	*Concerned person (who will take responsibility for the solution?)*
William	William
Problem behaviour:	*Objective (changed behaviour):*
Has been thinking about killing himself	Will keep himself safe
Context or setting:	*Context or setting:*
In his flat	In his flat and outside
Time frame(s):	*Time frame:*
Over the last week	Over the next three days

give a clear indication of the problem and strategies to help William keep himself safe. If William doesn't experience any improvement, each of the care plan's interventions can be reviewed. Is he following them, including attending appointments? Is he able to do what he'd planned to do? Is he taking his medication? Is he re-establishing his routine? Has anything happened that has worsened his thoughts or increased his stress? If any of these are a problem, the care plan can be adapted and, if necessary, more restrictive options explored.

The point of having William as the concerned person, both in 'owning' the problem and being responsible for the solution is not just about helping him with his recovery but also because, ultimately, he will be the only person able to keep himself safe, as evidenced by the fact that people manage to self-harm and kill themselves even when in hospital, including when a member of staff has been detailed to stay with the patient at all times, within arms' length (Appleby et al., 2006).

However, the clinicians are taking a very active role in supporting him with this. Their interventions mostly mirror his, e.g. meeting with him, looking at his list, helping him problem solve, calling his brother and giving him his medication on a daily basis initially. All these things are very directly linked to stopping him acting upon his suicidal thoughts and, hopefully, reducing those thoughts as well as allowing them to focus on the specific issues with which he is grappling.[ii]

The next example looks at how Oliver's risk management is organised in an inpatient setting, which would take place in a situation where he was only able to provide limited assurances of his ability to keep himself and others safe.

Example of a safety care plan written for a patient in an inpatient setting

Here, as seen in clinical example 23, Oliver has been able to describe his thoughts about Daniel and some of the nurses on the ward, how he feels about violence and his potential for assaulting those who he believes pose a threat to him. Again, this involves trying to capture Oliver's view of the world by acknowledging he doesn't feel safe, and writing the plan using Oliver's words as much as possible.

Problem:
For the last two days I haven't felt safe on the ward and have been thinking about hitting other people to protect myself.

Objective:
For the next week I will stay safe on the ward and not harm anyone else.

Interventions

I will:

1. Stay in a different part of the ward to Daniel, Ola and Jane at all times, including at medication times and meal times, when I will have my meals in my room.
2. Meet with one of my nurses for 5-10 minutes at the start of each shift to talk about how safe I feel, including what number I am at on my scale, and what I will do to remain safe.
3. Every two hours, practice the distraction techniques I use when I'm feeling stressed, like listening to music, doing deep breathing and the five senses exercise.[iii]
4. Once a day, for 15 minutes, talk with one of my nurses about why I feel unsafe and about what I'm thinking, as well as look at things I can do to help me stay safe.
5. Tell one of the nurses (I feel safe with) if I have moved up the scale to 6, so they are aware of the potential risk.
6. Tell the nurses and return to my room if I am having thoughts about hurting someone.
7. Acknowledge the nurse checking my safety every 15 minutes and, if I feel I'm unable to cope or might harm someone, tell the nurse and talk about what I'll do to stay safe.
8. Even though I don't want it, take the medication I've been prescribed.

My nurses will:

1. Make sure Daniel, Ola and Jane stay in a different part of the ward to me at all times, including at medication times and meal times, when a nurse (but not Ola or Jane) will bring my meals to me in my room.
2. Meet with me for 5–10 minutes at the start of each shift to talk about how safe I feel, including what number I am at on my scale, and what I will do to remain safe.
3. Remind me, every two hours, to practice my distraction techniques for when I'm feeling stressed, like listening to music, doing deep breathing and the five senses exercise.
4. Once a day, for 15 minutes, talk with me about why I feel unsafe and about what I'm thinking, as well as look at things I can do to help me stay safe. If I have moved up the scale to 6, talk with me about what I'll do to stay safe.
5. Make sure I return to my room if I am having thoughts about hurting someone.
6. Check on my safety every 15 minutes and, if I'm unable to cope or might harm someone, plan with me what I'll do to stay safe.
7. Even though I don't want it, give me the medication I've been prescribed and make sure I take it.

In this care plan, the formula is exactly the same as the one written for William. There is:

- A concerned person: *Oliver.*
- A defined problem: *he hasn't felt safe and has been thinking about hitting other people to protect himself.*
- A setting: *on the ward.*
- A time frame: *for the last two days.*

The clinical team view the primary cause of his potential violence to be his psychosis. But, by acknowledging that his current – and dangerous – behaviour is motivated by his anxiety about what others might do to him and his own perception of being unsafe, this enables the nurses to include in the objective a commitment to not hitting anyone else. Had that been listed as the sole objective, why would Oliver be motivated to try and meet that? In his 'world', that leaves him more vulnerable.

Again, the interventions are detailed but incorporate his own scale, using it as a direct mechanism to try and actively involve him in keeping others safe, as well as coping strategies he has described using.

Even though he has been quite dismissive of others and minimised his violence in earlier discussions with his nurse, the fact that he has been taken seriously, been enabled to articulate his experience in some detail and had that validated – without any collusion or agreement that this is what is *actually* happening – has formed the basis for a degree of mutual cooperation. The one thing he is not in agreement with is the need for medication, but the team have made it clear that he will have to take it and can be treated under the Mental Health Act if he refuses to take it voluntarily. At least at the time of discussion, he has reluctantly accepted this.

As with William's care plan, if there is not any progress, the interventions in Oliver's plan can be reviewed both for his concordance and their effectiveness, while also monitoring whether or not the nurses have been able to adhere to their commitments.

What is significantly different is that a decision has been made not to move Oliver to another ward but also not to move either Daniel, the named patient at risk of assault by Oliver. There have been several discussions with Daniel about the situation. He has said he wants to stay on the ward as he knows the team here and is hoping to be discharged soon. He has said he will cooperate with the plan by always staying in a different part of the ward from Oliver. The nurses Oliver has identified as 'doing things' to him have also agreed to stay on the ward. After discussion throughout the team and a careful review of the risk management plan and Oliver's current level of collaboration, it has been decided to proceed.

Key Clinical Tip

Care plans need to be:

- clear and focused on one issue;
- easy to understand;
- easy to access;
- used by the team, not just the person who wrote it;
- using a formula that translates from problem to objective;
- wherever possible, collaborative.

In addition to the written plan with Oliver, there is a broader risk management plan, including continency planning:

1. Oliver will be moved from the ward if there is an increase in the risk, he makes further threats or stops adhering to his care plan.
2. An additional nurse will be on the ward on every shift to manage the arrangements agreed with him about always staying in a different part of the ward to those he has threatened.

3. The nurses' rota has been reorganised so that Jane and Ola won't be working on the same shift, to give the nursing team the necessary flexibility during the shift.
4. Jane and Ola can be withdrawn from the ward at any time if it is felt unsafe for them to remain or they choose to move.
5. If Daniel does not continue to cooperate in maintaining his safety, e.g. by staying apart from Oliver, the nurse in charge of the shift in which this occurs will convene an emergency meeting of the team to discuss a revision to the plan, which might include transferring Daniel to another ward if Oliver has been making good progress.[iv]

A management plan for a patient who cannot or will not collaborate

As has been noted, there will be times when, despite the efforts of the clinical team, the patient either cannot or will not collaborate. When there are sufficient concerns about specific risks, this necessitates the team initiating a management plan (see Box 10).

Box 10:   Emma and a management plan

In this example, Emma has been attempting to work with the home treatment team but had a prolonged argument with her mother after her mother said she needed a larger financial contribution to the running of the house. Emma thought this unfair. She was further distressed when an old schoolfriend had not returned her calls or responded to messages left. Already feeling very stressed, Emma then became frustrated with different nurses visiting her. She said she was being deliberately messed around by nurses asking her the same questions on almost every visit, often then giving contradictory answers to her questions. When a nurse she had found particularly helpful didn't visit again, she asked if this was a deliberate attempt to destabilise her. Colleagues noted the nurse who responded to that question escalated the situation with defensive and emotion laden comments, which ended with Emma demanding they leave. Emma said the nurses only seemed interested in giving her medication and, despite promising an appointment with the consultant, that hadn't happened.

After three days of visits, she insisted she was no longer having any thoughts of harming herself. She then wasn't at home on three occasions when she had agreed to a visit and said she wanted to discharge herself from the team's care to wait to be seen by her regular care coordinator. This was agreed and she was discharged by the home treatment team.

Two days later, her mother brought her to the Emergency Department after she found Emma on the floor in the living room and difficult to rouse. Emma promptly vomited and revealed she had been storing up the anti-depressants prescribed for her and taken twelve Sertraline 100mg tablets, with ten Paracetamol 500mg tablets and six Promethazine 25mg tablets.

Emma was treated medically but, while waiting to be seen by the liaison psychiatry team, left the Department. Her mother went after her and found her at a nearby garage, extremely tearful and threatening to spray petrol from one of the pumps onto herself. Her mother persuaded her to go back to the hospital but, soon after they set off, Emma hit her mother, forcing her to stop the car. Emma ran off but was found by the police an hour later back at the bridge she had jumped from into the river a week earlier.

Brought back to the Emergency Department by the police, Emma said she didn't need help, there was nothing wrong with her and she had no intention of harming herself again. She would not discuss the self-poisoning incident, what happened at the garage or why she had returned to the bridge. Unable to agree a plan with Emma to help her remain safe, the liaison psychiatry team took the view that her actions were inconsistent from recent days when she had talked about, among other things, her desire to return to university and aspirations as a writer. Unconvinced she would be safe in the community, whatever support was offered, they decided it was their duty of care to respond to Emma's extreme distress. Viewing her behaviour as a disturbed form of engagement rather than an attempt to disengage and, given the immediate risk of Emma either ending her life or seriously harming herself, and evidence she was lacking capacity, the team concluded it was in her best interests to detain her under Section Two of the Mental Health Act.

Within minutes of arriving on the acute admission ward, Emma tried to leave. She either sat mutely or demanded she be allowed to go. When told she couldn't leave, she said she was being driven mad by staff and they were forcing her to hurt herself. She said she would cut herself or tie a ligature and strangle herself. Soon after, she found a small glass bottle of perfume in another patient's bedroom and broke this with the intention of cutting her face and was restrained by three nurses to prevent her from doing so.

As she was unable to engage in developing a care plan, a management plan was written by her primary nurse in collaboration with the nurse in charge of the shift.

In this example, the route by which the inpatient clinical team needed to write a management plan has not been without its problems. Issues have arisen due to organisational structures, e.g. the model by which home treatment teams send different staff to visit someone who needs consistency and continuity of care. There are further complications with the responses of individual staff members, all compounding the challenge of working with Emma when she is in such a heightened state.

A management plan differs from a care plan in that it is written in the third person i.e. about Emma. There are no interventions for her; all the interventions identified are for the staff team. An essential element, as well as working to try to stop her from harming herself, are constant attempts to engage with her and assess her ability to work with the team and begin a collaborative relationship. The management plan in this case reads as follows:

Problem:
Since arriving on the ward, Emma has made specific threats to end her life, attempted to cut her throat and cannot yet work with staff to help her remain safe.

Objective:
Over the next three days, the ward team will try to maintain Emma's safety on the ward.

Team interventions on the ward:

1. Ensure Emma remains on the ward and always has a nurse within eyesight, so she can ask for support at any time and receive an immediate response, as well as attempting to prevent any further self-harm or suicide attempt.
2. The nurse staying within eyesight of Emma will try to negotiate how she wants to spend that time but remind her they won't be talking about her previous suicide attempts or self-harming behaviour because that will be addressed by her primary and associate nurses.
3. Encourage Emma to take part in low stimuli activity on the ward when she is able, particularly trying to distract her from her intrusive thoughts about hurting herself and ending her life.
4. Encourage relaxation techniques every two hours as Emma has previously said these help her.
5. If Emma is overstimulated by being with other patients or her own distress, to encourage her to spend time in the quiet room or her own bedroom.
6. Fully re-assess Emma's safety each shift, based on what she says, her behaviour and ability to reach agreement with nursing staff. This is to be repeated if specific changes are noted that might increase risk.
7. Give Emma a 15 minute period each day when she can spend time with her primary or associate nurses to talk specifically about her safety on the ward and what happened that led to her being admitted.
8. In addition, they will ask about anything that has been helpful on the ward, and anything she thinks we can do that would be helpful.
9. If she becomes very unsettled, quietly talk with him about things that help her feel calm and in control and try and resolve external issues that might have caused a problem.
10. Administer her routine medication as prescribed (ensuring she takes it) and PRN medication if she asks for it or a decision is made that she would benefit from it in a potential crisis.

Table 5.3 Structuring a management plan

Identifying the problem	Setting an objective to resolve the problem
Concerned person (whose problem is it?)	*Concerned person (who will take responsibility for the solution?)*
Emma	The ward team
Problem behaviour: Made specific threats to end her life, attempted to cut her throat and cannot agree to work with staff to help her remain safe	*Objective (changed behaviour):* Try to maintain Emma's safety
Context or setting: The ward	*Context or setting:* The ward
Time frame(s): Since arriving	*Time frame:* Over the next three days

A number of clear interventions are in place to in order to try and keep Emma safe, provide containment and reduce the internal and external stimuli she experiences as these are likely to be exacerbating her distress, ruminations and thoughts of self-harm/suicide.

There are several reasons the nurses providing ongoing support will not be talking with her about her self-harming and suicidal experiences but leaving that to her primary nurses. It could be potentially overwhelming for Emma to have to talk about this with different people at unplanned times during the day without any structure. There would be the potential for staff to give inconsistent if not contradictory responses, which will likely escalate her disturbance and introduce the potential for divergent views about her within the team. This, in turn, could increase the risk for Emma.

Because of the need for consistency and continuity of care, there are several things an incoming shift team would have to be aware of. Those managing the shift therefore need to ensure the plan is communicated thoroughly to everyone working, even having paper copies available for them to read, going through it thoroughly at each shift handover and with a specific briefing for those nurses who would be staying within eyesight and providing immediate support for Emma.

Although the plan runs for three days before a multi-professional team review, it would be necessary for the nursing staff to review it on a shift-by-shift basis and adjust the interventions *where necessary*, because responding to change needs to be balanced by maintaining consistency, not reacting to either slight progress or minor setbacks only to reverse the changes within a few hours. The plan also makes allowance for every attempt to engage with Emma and seek her collaboration.

From the clinician's perspective, this is about establishing clear boundaries and providing a safe and containing environment. At this time, Emma may well experience this as wrongfully being deprived of her liberty, punitive and alienating. It should also be remembered that it can be frightening and frustrating, even for an individual whose outward behaviour is perceived as 'hostile' and 'challenging'. Emma's desire to harm herself has meaning for her, it is a means for attempting to manage unmanageable distress and she is being thwarted in that. There is often a concern that imposing restrictions in this way might 'damage' the relationship with the patient. That is a risk but, when it is concluded that it is the only safe way to manage specific, serious and immediate risks without the collaboration of the person when that person lacks capacity, that in itself has to figure in the risk management process. In the short term, clearly, concisely and honestly communicating what is being done and why, using de-escalation skills and trying to keep the environment around the patient as calm as possible, is often the best that can be done, though it is impossible to emphasise enough the importance of consistency and boundaries conveyed in as compassionate a way as possible.

It will almost certainly take some time to effect improvements in the person's mental state or how they perceive what is happening. Certainly, you cannot reassure them that things are 'all right'. Nor are they likely to agree to any attempts you make to 'get them' to 'calm down'. However, as much about their situation as possible should be stabilised. Your calmness, consistency and confidence in what you are doing can be very containing (Casement, 1985). You can also affect the environment and minimise the stimulation around them to maintain the physical safety of the patient and others (Hart, 2013b).

Inpatient nurses should not shy away from providing these important nursing treatments, and proactively intervening. Indeed, what is often termed, and delivered as, enhanced observation can be re-thought of as enhanced personal support. The change is not about semantics. It is about a different approach. Rather than a nurse being allocated to 'do the observations' (often with no briefing beforehand and not even being sure what they are supposed to be looking for), it involves nurses being allocated to the patient's immediate care and available to the patient throughout that allocated period – as opposed to their primary and associate nurses, who maintain a relationship with them as they would with any other patient – proactively and consistently working to a care plan that is geared towards specific risk management interventions (Onyenaobiya and Hart, 2013).

Clinical Example 25:   Responding to challenging behaviour when managing serious risk

Emma has been shouting on the ward and is being seen by her primary nurse.

Emma: [*Shouts*] I want to go. [*More quietly*] The doctor in A&E said I'd be reviewed when I arrived here, and I wouldn't have to stay.

Clinician: I'm not sure about what the doctor said to you in the A&E Department–

Emma: [*Interrupts*] You should. It's your job.

Clinician: I have heard–

Emma: [*Interrupts*] Look it up.

Clinician: I'm not sure what you mean.

Emma: Why not?

Clinician: I've heard what you've said about how hard it is for you to be here but, to try to help you through this crisis, the doctors thought it necessary for you to be detained under the Mental Health Act–

Emma: [*Interrupts*] It's not helping.

Clinician: I know we disagree about you being here, but I want to help you.

Emma: Then let me go home. There are things I need to sort out now or else I'm going to lose my university place for good. Think that's going to help me? Really? I'm not going to hurt myself, if that's what you're worried about.

Clinician: That's what you told the home treatment team a few days ago. But then you made a serious attempt to end your life. Today, you were at a garage and talking about setting yourself alight. I can't see what has changed since.

Emma: I'm okay now.

Clinician: You say that but you've looked very distressed since you arrived.

Emma: Whatever you say. [*Silence*] You're just making things worse. I will harm myself if I have to stay.

Clinician: I want to help you leave here as quickly as possible. Everyone in the team does. I know that when things are difficult for you, hurting yourself seems to help and it must seem odd to say I'm keeping you here to help you be safe when it's so stressful–

Emma:	[*Shouts*] Then let me go!
Clinician:	As a team, we're agreed about this, Emma. We need to see you can keep yourself safe here, and not harm yourself, before even thinking about you leaving.
Emma:	I told you. I'm safe. Right?
Clinician:	I don't think you're able to say that now and be confident it won't change.
Emma:	So, you're calling me a liar.
Clinician:	No. I'm saying that I'm concerned that, if you had the opportunity, or could see no other way out of your situation, you might try again to kill yourself.
Emma:	You're treating me like a little kid.
Clinician:	I'm sorry it feels like that. It's not my intention.
Emma:	What are you going to do then?
Clinician:	You have a copy of the plan. We'll keep on with that until we – you, and us as a team – can agree on a change that puts you more in charge of things.
Emma:	How long does this have to go on?
Clinician:	Let's see if we can get through the rest of this shift, shall we? That will be nine o'clock tonight.
Emma:	What then? I don't want some idiot looking me up and down all day and all night like I'm a freak.
Clinician:	Then we plan for the night. But the nurses are not there for that. They're there for you, if and when you need some support. You can negotiate how that happens.
Emma:	Why can't you do it?
Clinician:	I'll meet with you as close to four o'clock as I can, for 15 minutes, like it says in the plan.
Emma:	Waste of time. [*Returns to her room and lies on her bed*]

The clinician here is absolutely clear and direct in her communication, expressing the exact nature of her concerns, why she has them and what she is doing as a consequence, always linking this back to team decisions and the plan that is now in place. She recognises and acknowledges both the areas of disagreement and the impact it has on Emma, empathises but does not allow Emma's distress or criticisms to cloud her clinical judgement. When Emma asks if the nurse is calling her a liar, rather than 'defend' herself or get into a 'yes/no' discussion, the nurse simply reminds Emma of things she has already said that have led the nurse to her conclusion.

Behaving in a consistent, clear and compassionate fashion, alongside the other communication skills required when having to go against the wishes of the patient in a particularly challenging situation, will do as much as anything to 'contain' the patient's emotions and assist in trying to maintain a relationship with the patient that has its basis in being helpful, genuine and honest.

> **Key clinical tip**
>
> The five 'C's helps **contain** the patient's distress when you're going against their wishes in exerting your **clinical** judgement in a challenging situation.
>
> Communicate in a way that is:
>
> 1. Consistent.
> 2. Clear.
> 3. Compassionate.
> 4. Concise.
> 5. Caring.

Risk management that is proactive and enabling

A lot of risk management is reactive – being enacted in response to something potentially dangerous the patient is doing. This often involves restrictions placed upon the person, i.e. interventions designed to stop something happening. However, as the person's clinical presentation improves, different techniques come into play where the patient and clinician agree to make the interventions less reactive or expose the patient to more potential risk because it is believed they are now able to manage that for themselves more effectively. This may involve making the environment less restrictive. At its most extreme this might mean coming out of seclusion and back into the ward environment, graduating from escorted to unescorted leave from an inpatient unit, or being discharged. In a community setting it might be that daily visits are reduced to once every two or three days. It might involve returning to work or a situation that was previously very stressful or potentially triggering and where the risk was previously deemed too unsafe.

This process has often been termed therapeutic risk management or positive risk management. Risk management should always be therapeutic and positive but a term is required to highlight the shift from being restrictive and/or preventative to something more empowering, hence using the term 'enabling'.

Enabling risk management is very different from taking risks without the clinicians involved having seriously thought about the issues or discussed them with the patient. Enabling risk taking is deciding upon a plan of action which does have recognised associated risks but where the potential benefits have been assessed as outweighing the potential negative consequences of the plan. An example of this is agreeing with William that he will remain in his flat and be seen daily after being assessed, having seriously considered ending his life while in an emotionally distressed state. The risk is far from eliminated at this stage but this approach is judged to be more beneficial than admitting him into an acute ward against his will in that it:

- allows him to maintain a degree of manageable responsibility for his safety;
- builds upon his coping strategies in the environment where they are required;
- assists the team in engaging with him;
- takes advantage of his collaboration in his risk management.

It also means that the potentially negative experience of being on a psychiatric ward is avoided although, as noted above, anxiety about the impact on the team's relationship with the patient should not be the defining reason for taking a less restrictive option. That should always be governed by risk.

Enabling risk management can only take place in the context of a robust risk assessment and risk management plan, taking into account advance directives (where these are in place), an exploration of 'what if?' scenarios and contingency plans. It is reliant upon having developed, with the patient, a shared understanding of, and openly acknowledging, the potential risks to the patient of their own behaviours, the triggers and drivers for these behaviours. The negative consequences of those behaviours, were they carried out, need to be balanced against the positive benefits of the use of agreed, adaptive coping mechanisms to combat them. Focussing on the strengths of the patient and their social network, it offers the opportunity for the person to drive their own recovery with others' help (see Box 11).

It's not just the clinician(s) working directly with the patient who need to agree this process, but also the rest of the team and anyone indirectly involved. Consistent and regular supervision should be used to provide opportunities to discuss and reflect on potential decisions. Detailed checks are required on what is safe, what is possible and what actual risks are being addressed all of which should be discussed in clinical reviews.

The underlying principles of enabling risk management are that clinical decisions should always be:

- defensible rather than defensive;
- in the best interests of the patient;
- seeking to provide the least restrictive options in terms of their care.

Box 11:   A checklist for teams and patients when working with enabling risk management

1. What needs to, and can, change?
2. Are you clear about the patient's experiences and understanding of risk?
3. Are you clear about the carer experience and understanding of risk (primarily, are they happy about the particular risks to be taken and any responsibility that may be placed upon them)?
4. Have you clearly defined potential risks and their context?
5. Is everyone clear about the planned stages for the proposed changes?
6. Has there been a clear articulation of the desired outcomes?
7. Has there been a clear identification of strengths and coping mechanisms?
8. Has there been an estimate of what could go wrong, the estimated likelihood of this happening and potential worst outcomes?
9. What potential safety nets are in place, including identification of early warning signs linked to a crisis and contingency plan?
10. Have you and the patient explored the 'what if' scenarios?
11. What was the outcome of previous attempt(s) at this course of action?
12. How was it managed, and what will now be done differently?

13. How will progress be monitored?
14. Who agrees to the approach (and who disagrees?)
15. When will it be reviewed? (O'Brien and Hart, 2013.)

Relapse profiles and crisis plans

If you and your team have been involved in caring for, and treating, someone who has been through a crisis, it is always useful to evaluate with them what happened during that period and, even more importantly, the events that led up to it. From such a discussion two things can be developed that will be useful in the event of a change in the person's circumstances that could lead to a further crisis. The first is a relapse profile. There are different models for this, some involving work with the individual concerned and others that explore relapse prevention and self-monitoring from the perspectives of the patient, family and staff (Gamble and Curthoys, 2004). The example below (Table 5.4) involves looking at the events that occurred, and their impact on the person's mental health. This is often a painful and difficult process for the person. There may be elements of the story they

Table 5.4 A sample relapse profile using William's case study

Thoughts	Feelings	Behaviour
Kelly is fed up with me. She thinks I'm not a good partner and can't provide for her.	Misunderstood and anxious.	Compensate by doing things I think will please Kelly.
This is too hard. I'm not getting anywhere. Kelly's angry and getting at me. What's coming next?	More anxious. Frustrated.	Stay in. Do less. Try to avoid Kelly but argue because she's angry with me.
Worry about things that have happened, especially Dad's illness and his death. Why did I say or do that? People must think I'm an idiot. What will go wrong tomorrow?	Tired. Irritable.	Can't sleep. Try to communicate how I'm feeling but find myself complaining and arguing even more. Stop having sex.
Kelly is going to leave me. Things will go wrong. I can't pay my bills. I'm going to lose the flat. I let my dad down. I should have done more. How will I get through the day?	Abandoned and 'lost' but also alone and resentful. Guilty.	Stop going out. Spend more time on my own. Stay in bed. Don't answer the phone.
Everyone thinks I can't cope and I'm weak. No one understands or wants me around. People blame me for everything. I should hurt myself. It might make this go away.	Really miserable. Exhausted. Don't feel hungry. Don't feel like doing anything. Ashamed.	Eat less. Drink more alcohol. Sleep less. Wake up early. Avoid people. Don't want to talk to anyone.
There's no way out of this, no answer to my problems. It's all my fault. Everyone would be better off if I wasn't here. I'd be better off dead. How would I kill myself?	Trapped, boxed in. Stuck. Suffocating. Angry. Really angry.	Withdraw even more. Drinking more. Pacing around. Maybe scraping knife across my skin. Go and get tablets.
I can't take any more. I have to kill myself.	There's no way to describe how I feel.	Take tablets.

now find embarrassing, and it is natural for a patient to want to minimise some parts of it. However, it is incumbent upon the clinician to help them overcome this and work through the story in detail, possibly even reminding them of some of elements of it, if they are going to make proper sense of it and incorporate them into a plan to prevent it happening again.

It is broken into three components: thoughts, feelings and behaviour. The person may need assistance in differentiating thoughts from feelings. It shouldn't be presumed that the person is experienced in articulating feelings, and they may need assistance with this. To help them, it might be useful to explain that thoughts can be spoken aloud, e.g. "They're after me," or "I'm not good at this." For the purposes of this exercise, the words 'I feel...' would presage the emotional state that follows e.g. "I feel anxious," or "I feel happy."

Drawing up something like this with the person is a helpful way for both of you to understand the process, piece by piece, by which the original crisis came about. In doing this you can also help the person identify warning signs of when things might be recurring, or that they are relapsing. Even if there are significant changes in the person's experience, as is the case with William, where he has separated from his partner, he can look back on the pattern of his thoughts, how they relate to his feelings and how both affect his behaviour.

This exercise might need a number of sessions to allow the person the opportunity to reflect and help them with some painful feelings. But they can then think about the second part of the process, a crisis plan to try and prevent a relapse (Hillard and Zitek, 2004). This can be formatted into a plan in much the same way you would an immediate risk management plan.

Steps to help William prevent a crisis:

1. Keep my daily routine going, even if I'm not working.
2. Make sure I eat regularly (and not too late and not too many takeaways).
3. Sleep at least seven hours a night and don't nap during the day.
4. Exercise every day, even if it's going for regular walks, but preferably attending yoga classes and playing football with my mates.
5. Set myself daily tasks and keep to my plans.
6. Visit my brother and Mum once a week, let them know how I'm feeling and get feedback from them about what they see me doing.
7. Start looking for work but if I can't find anything remind myself that I can look for something else.
8. Don't drink alcohol while I'm taking anti-depressants.
9. Keep meeting with my nurse as arranged.
10. Keep a check on where I am on my mood scale and alert family and my nurse if I'm slipping down it.

If I start to become anxious and miserable or thinking about harming myself:

1. Check my list of things to prevent a crisis and see if I'm doing everything – if not, try and do it.
2. Challenge any negative thoughts. Remind myself I don't normally think like this.
3. Check things out with people I know, e.g. what they're thinking, how they feel towards me, without them thinking I'm weird or leaving me feeling silly.
4. Do routine deep breathing and relaxation exercises four times a day and when I'm starting to feel more anxious than usual.

5. If things get worse, contact the community mental health team and ask for an urgent appointment.
6. If I have an unexpected crisis, ring the crisis helpline or go to the A&E Department.

The more closely linked a crisis management plan is to the work that went into assessing and managing the risk originally, the more likely they are to be successful. However, one of the problems arising out of fragmented services is that clinicians working with the patient may never have seen them in a crisis, have no idea how the person was affected when their situation was at its worst and, consequently, little understanding of how to develop a plan to avoid a further crisis. In a worst case scenario, a patient may have been seen in crisis first by a liaison psychiatry team, then a crisis team and finally a home treatment team (with the possibility of an inpatient team somewhere in that mix) before being passed onto a locality based community team. If this was the case the clinician responsible for trying to help prevent a relapse will need to undertake a careful scanning of the patient's records as well as conduct an in depth interview to gain the patient's perspective on the story of the development of the crisis.

Record keeping and good documentation

Good record keeping is an integral part of risk management. As has been noted throughout the *Pocket Guide*, risk management follows on from the risk formulation that resulted from the risk assessment and everything written about it should be seen as directly linked. It should be comprehensive, written in such a way that anyone can understand it and accessible to those who need to see it.

Everything recorded should be relevant, as objective as possible and avoid descriptive labels and terms such as 'angry', 'violent', 'dangerous', which can be highly subjective, when describing an act that has taken place, e.g. 'Oliver was shouting loudly, swearing and making threats to staff. He then threw a chair across the room at Staff Nurse Murray which narrowly missed her legs', or 'Oliver shouted at Nurse Murray, saying that he would hit her if she did not leave the room but walked away without any intervention'.

If generic terms such as 'anger' or 'violence' have to be used, the clinician should be as precise and accurate as possible when communicating with others, either orally or in documentation, with the writer also acknowledging that this is their opinion, e.g. 'Oliver appeared angry, threatening violence and I was of the impression he would act upon his threats unless we withdrew'.

It is important to differentiate between fact and opinion. It may be a fact that Emma took a large number of tablets. The intent may not be clear, and she may be saying afterwards that she did not intend to kill herself. You should not write down your own ideas about her intentions as if they are fact. Rather, indicate your subjective impression, e.g.:

Emma's mother reported her daughter took 30 Sertraline 100mg tablets, with ten Paracetamol 500mg tablets and six Promethazine 25mg tablets last night at approximately 21.00hrs. Although Emma now states she did not intend to kill herself, it is my impression that she wanted to die and was disappointed to have survived the self poisoning. This is based on her mother's account of what she had been saying in the days leading up to the incident and when she first found her after the overdose.

If you need to make a lengthy entry, it is useful to use sub headings to signpost the reader to the different elements of what you've written. For example, if writing an account of Emma's admission to the acute inpatient unit and events leading up to a management plan being initiated, the sub headings might be:

- Reason for admission
- Emma's arrival on the ward
- Attempts to leave the ward
- Discussions with Emma about her safety
- Emma's current risk on the ward
- Decision to initiate a management plan

If making an entry into a risk assessment section on an electronic records system that does not automatically record the location, date and time, these should always be added.

It is also important to remember anything you record will be open to a wider audience, so ensure your entry is unambiguous and conveys the information you want it to.

Box 12:   Ten tips for good record keeping

1. Remember, your entry will be read by a wider audience, so it needs to be:
   - as brief as possible, but include all relevant details;
   - clearly written;
   - if the entry is lengthy, think about using subheadings to signpost the reader to important sections.
2. Write your entry so that someone reading it can understand what you mean and act upon any instructions for clinicians on the next shift/next day etc.
3. Avoid language that doesn't actually convey what has been happening, e.g. terms like 'unsettled' or 'threatening'. Explain what the person was doing and saying and exactly what you have observed. Avoid phrases such as 'settled in mood and mental state'. They are meaningless. What is the person's mood? Only write about their mental state if you have assessed it. If referring to their behaviour, describe that. Rather than 'slept well', state how many hours they appear to have slept.
4. Where there are clinical decisions made, e.g. changes in prescribed observations, explain the reasons for your decisions.
5. Describe the events that led to an incident. An extra sentence can be like gold dust in helping the reader understand what happened and, importantly, why it happened.
6. Do not make personal comments in your entries that may be insulting or unnecessarily distressing to the person should they have access to their records. However, do not censor what needs to be written and be explicit about risk and other important issues. The important thing is to ensure it is written professionally and evidenced by being fact-based or an impression drawn from a valid hypothesis (see below).

7. When you are expressing your impression or 'feeling' about a risk, you should clearly state this, differentiating it from fact-based evidence e.g. 'Emma states she will not harm herself but, based on her behaviour and other things she has said in the past few hours, I think it likely she would hurt herself if distressed and she had the opportunity'.

8. Record what you explained to the patient, i.e. their rights under the Mental Health Act. Also, if someone lacks capacity to make a safety care plan, make sure this is recorded.

9. Being explicit about key questions you have asked during a risk assessment can be useful in communicating how the information emerged during the interview.

10. Your entries should be recorded within the span of your duty or, if in a crisis, at the earliest opportunity and no later than first thing the following day. If you don't have the time or opportunity to write a full account of what has happened, ensure that what is most important is recorded, with a note to explain why you couldn't complete it and when that will happen (O'Brien and Hart, 2013).

Notes

i This is more complex in a prison setting, where non compliance due to mental health problems or in the case of someone who is suicidal will almost certainly necessitate the involvement of discipline staff. In the case of risk to self, officers will lead the ACCT process and possibly initiate constant observation. If the risk is to others, even if this is related to an individual's mental health, it may require restraint and moving the person into an inpatient unit wherever possible. Healthcare staff will, however, have a crucial role in supporting prison staff and trying to work with the person. This is when multi professional working has to be at its most effective and joint care plans i.e. highlighting interventions by officers and healthcare staff an essential element.

ii For nurses involved in this process, there is a secondary benefit, in that this kind of active work, not just in William's care but also his treatment, gives the nurse a clearer role and greater degree of authority to go with the responsibility they often have.

iii This involves the person noting, in the present, five things they can see, four things they can touch, three things they can hear, two things they can smell and one thing they can taste.

iv The actual case on which Oliver's character and scenario is based was managed in a very similar way to that described here and the outcome was very positive. He gradually realised the people he was concerned about weren't doing any of the things he believed and, without him having to resort to violence, he could remain safe. Taking his medication as prescribed lessened his psychotic phenomena and his perception of his situation changed, contributing to changed relationships with the clinical team and his eventual step down from a medium secure unit to low secure setting and ultimate discharge to the community after several years in hospital.

References and selected bibliography

Appleby, L., Shaw, J., Kapur, N., Windfuhr, K., Ashton, A., Swinson, N. and While, D. (2006) *Avoidable Deaths: Five Year Report by the National Confidential Inquiry into Suicide and Homicide By People with Mental Illness*. Manchester: University of Manchester.

Ayre, K., Owen, G.S. and Moran, P. (2017) Mental capacity and borderline personality disorder. *BJPsych Bulletin*, 41, 33–36. DOI: 10.1192/pb.bp.115.052753.

Bennewith, O., Gunnell, D., Peters, T.J. Hawton, K. and House, A. (2004) Variations in the hospital management of self-harm in adults in England: observational study. *British Medical Journal*, 328, 1108–1109.

Breeze, J.A. and Repper, J. (1998) Struggling for control: the care experiences of 'difficult' patients in mental health services. *Journal of Advanced Nursing*, 28, 1301–1311.

Casement, P. (1985) *On Learning From the Patient*. London: Routledge.

Department of Health (2005) Mental Capacity Act. London: Department of Health.

Department of Health (2010) *See, Think, Act: Your Guide to Relational Security*. London: Department of Health.

Doyle, M. and Dolan, M. (2006). Predicting community violence from patients discharged from mental health services. *British Journal of Psychiatry*, 189, 520–526.

Gamble, C. and Curthoys, J. (2004) Psychosocial Interventions. In: Norman, I. and

Ryrie, I. (eds.) *The Art and Science of Mental Health Nursing: a textbook of principles and practice*. Oxford: Oxford University Press.

Hart, C. (2013a) *Working Effectively as a Primary Nurse*. London: South West London & St George's Mental Health NHS Trust.

Hart, C. (2013b) *The SAFE Model of Nursing in a Psychiatric Intensive Care Unit*. London: South West London & St George's Mental Health NHS Trust.

Hillard, R. and Zitek, B. (2004) *Emergency Psychiatry*. New York: McGraw-Hill.

Maden, T. (2007) *Treating violence: a guide to risk management in mental health*. Oxford University Press: Oxford.

O'Brien, J. and Hart, C. (2013) *Clinical Risk Assessment and Risk Management*. London: South West London & St George's Mental Health NHS Trust.

Onyenaobiya, A. and Hart, C. (2013) Intensive Personal Support as an Alternative to Enhanced Observations. Unpublished Paper.

Ritter, S. (1989) *Bethlem Royal and Maudsley Hospital Manual of Clinical Psychiatric Nursing Principles and Procedures*. London: HarperCollins.

Van Heeringen, C. and Maruia, A. (2003) Understanding the suicidal brain. *The British Journal of Psychiatry*, 183, 282–284.

Wheeler, M. (2012) *Law, Ethics and Professional Issues for Nursing*. London: Routledge.

Williams, J.M.G., Crane, C., Barnhofer, T. and Duggan, D. (2005) Psychology and suicidal behaviour: elaborating the entrapment model. In: Hawton, K. (ed.) *Prevention and Treatment of Suicidal Behaviour: from science to practice*. Oxford: Oxford University Press.

Summary and conclusions

This *Pocket Guide* has detailed the key issues about the practice of risk assessment and risk management in the area of mental health. Nonetheless, as was stated in the introduction, it has not set out to cover the entire evidence base or theory behind such practice and these are areas of knowledge that you should explore further. It is a rewarding area of study, which requires continual application given the changing evidence base and advances in knowledge. Moreover, the public rightly expect those clinicians involved in risk assessment and management in mental health to have the necessary expertise and skills to do this as effectively as possible.

Gaining that expertise and skill, however, requires practice and although this needs to take place under close supervision initially, it will only occur through the application of your experience and knowledge in clinical situations. In other words, there is no substitute for *doing*. As has been noted in the substantive text, as clinicians we can only ever minimise risk, not eliminate it. The complexity and difficulty of this work means, whether you perceive yourself as being at the novice or expert end of the spectrum, you won't always get it right, nor know everything about the patient and the risks they face. Never be afraid to ask for help and make good use of reflective practice and clinical supervision.

The statistics in Part 2 are there for your reference and highlight some important information and clinical risk factors. These cannot be used, however, as an alternative for a comprehensive assessment of the individual sitting in the room with you. The lists, tables and information boxes are not there to be 'ticked off' during an assessment but to be used as prompts, to provide a framework and structure for the assessment. Hopefully, both they and the clinical examples will stimulate your curiosity and willingness to carefully listen and think, helping you phrase your next question from an informed perspective but still based on what you have just heard the person say.

To quote an old and dear friend, always think about 'need to know and nice to know'. You have limited time, so make sure you have gained the essential information from the assessment to enable you to come up with the best possible risk management plan. If you're aware that you haven't got that yet, plan how you will make sufficient time and what contingency plan is required until you have. Again, as you near the end of an assessment, quoting another dear and old friend, ask yourself what you *don't* yet know about this person and always check if they have anything they still want to tell you that is important and relevant to the risk or potential risk.

Finally, a last reminder to emphasise that even the most robust assessment and management of risk cannot always prevent tragedies. Delving into all areas of risk, hoping for the best and planning for the worst, will allow you to manage those most obvious.

DOI: 10.4324/9781003171614-7

Careful consideration of those 'what if...?' questions will help you plan for the less obvious. Nonetheless, something may happen to change the situation in ways impossible to predict, even if that is only a change in the person's thinking, and lead to a serious incident or even the person's death. Reviewing such an event, you may at least be able to take comfort from seeing you had done the best job possible and that the risk was genuinely unforeseen. This is very different from someone repeating a past act or following the logical conclusions of past events or things they had been threatening, without there being an adequate plan in place to address it.

While you will always seek to collaborate with the person and work with their agenda as much as possible, don't be afraid to act in the best interests of the person when necessary, even if they disagree with you. Risk management, in all the details of its specific interventions, is a treatment and everyone has a right to treatment, even if they are arguing at the time that they don't want it. The risk management plan should not be driven by available resource but the needs of the person with you. That is an essential part of your duty of care. Once risk has been identified, a coherent, reasoned plan to assess it must be put in place.

Hopefully, the clinical examples will help you think about and find your own voice and use it. Each patient will teach you not only about themselves but also about the assessment process itself. What cannot be captured on the page are the moments you listen, look, think and then act, always in the interest of that person and any others who may be at risk as a consequence of that person's actions.

Index

Note: **Bold** page numbers refer to tables; *italic* page numbers refer to figures and page numbers followed by "n" denote endnotes.